Elisabeth Veronika Aichner

Skin grafting for donor site wounds in elderly patients

AF138596

Elisabeth Veronika Aichner

Skin grafting for donor site wounds in elderly patients

A prospective clinical trial comparing three different dressing materials in split-thickness skin graft surgery

Human Sciences Series

Impressum / Imprint
Bibliografische Information der Deutschen Nationalbibliothek: Die Deutsche Nationalbibliothek verzeichnet diese Publikation in der Deutschen Nationalbibliografie; detaillierte bibliografische Daten sind im Internet über http://dnb.d-nb.de abrufbar.
Alle in diesem Buch genannten Marken und Produktnamen unterliegen warenzeichen-, marken- oder patentrechtlichem Schutz bzw. sind Warenzeichen oder eingetragene Warenzeichen der jeweiligen Inhaber. Die Wiedergabe von Marken, Produktnamen, Gebrauchsnamen, Handelsnamen, Warenbezeichnungen u.s.w. in diesem Werk berechtigt auch ohne besondere Kennzeichnung nicht zu der Annahme, dass solche Namen im Sinne der Warenzeichen- und Markenschutzgesetzgebung als frei zu betrachten wären und daher von jedermann benutzt werden dürften.

Bibliographic information published by the Deutsche Nationalbibliothek: The Deutsche Nationalbibliothek lists this publication in the Deutsche Nationalbibliografie; detailed bibliographic data are available in the Internet at http://dnb.d-nb.de.
Any brand names and product names mentioned in this book are subject to trademark, brand or patent protection and are trademarks or registered trademarks of their respective holders. The use of brand names, product names, common names, trade names, product descriptions etc. even without a particular marking in this work is in no way to be construed to mean that such names may be regarded as unrestricted in respect of trademark and brand protection legislation and could thus be used by anyone.

Coverbild / Cover image: www.ingimage.com

Verlag / Publisher:
AV Akademikerverlag
ist ein Imprint der / is a trademark of
OmniScriptum GmbH & Co. KG
Heinrich-Böcking-Str. 6-8, 66121 Saarbrücken, Deutschland / Germany
Email: info@akademikerverlag.de

Herstellung: siehe letzte Seite /
Printed at: see last page
ISBN: 978-3-639-47620-0

Acknowledgement

First, I would like to thank my supervisors, Ass. Dr. Daryousch Parvizi and Univ. Prof. Dr. Lars-Peter Kamolz, for their guidance and for giving me helpful advice, as well as for granting me independence, while supporting me when necessary, and for their interest in helping me to achieve a quality study.

In addition, I am grateful to the whole medical and nursing staff of the Division of Plastic, Aesthetic and Reconstructive Surgery at the Medical University of Graz for their cooperation and assistance, for giving me advice and for always having patience in answering my questions. Of course, I would also like to thank every patient who made this study possible. In addition, I would like to express my gratitude to the photographers, Mrs. Andrea Maurer and Mr. Martin Stelzer, for their friendliness, their helpfulness and their untiring accessibility.

I am grateful to my whole family for constantly supporting me and for giving me helpful hands when I needed them; and for my important family of friends, like Martina, Thomas, Romana and Melanie who have always been there for me.

And finally I want to thank my little son for showing me the magic and beauty of life every day and for encouraging me to always try again to do well in being a small part of a very big meaningful whole.

Table of Contents

Abbreviations

AD	Anno Domini
ASA Score	American Society of Anesthesiologists Score
BC	Before Christ
bFGF	Basic fibroblast growth factor
Biatain Ibu	Biatain dressing saturated with ibuprofen
ECM	Extra cellular matrix
EGF	Epidermal growth factor
FGF	Fibroblast growth factor
FTSG	Full-thickness skin graft
GVHD	Graft versus host disease
HB-EGF	Heparin-binding epidermal growth factor
HWES	Hollander Wound Evaluation Scale
IGF-1	Insulin-like growth factor-1
Mepilex Ag	Polyurethane foam containing a silver salt
MRSA	Multiresistant Staphylococcus aureus
MWH	Moist wound healing
NSAIDs	Non-steroidal anti-inflammatory drugs
STSG	Split-thickness skin graft
PDGF	Platelet derived growth factor
p.s.	Sanatio per secundam intentionem
p.p.	Sanatio per primam intentionem
TGF-a	Transforming growth factor alpha
TGF-ß	Transforming growth factor beta
VAS	Visual Analogue Scale
VASm	Visual Analogue Scale in movement
VASr	Visual Analogue Scale at rest
VRE	Vancomycin resistant Enterococcus

ABSTRACT

Background: Skin grafting is a well-established procedure using skin or skin substitute to cover non-healing wounds or burns. Management of donor site wounds with a suitable dressing material in high-risk patient groups is crucial. These wounds are often painful for patients and can be infected as healing time especially in patients with comorbidities like diabetes or hypertension can be prolonged.

Methods: The aim of this study was to compare three different dressing materials in donor site wounds in a prospective clinical trial in a patient cohort aged 55 or older with one or more comorbidities. The grafts were harvested in a standardized procedure and wounds were dressed under sterile conditions with Biatain Ibu, Mepilex Ag or Suprathel. Dressing changes were scheduled day 10 to 14 when re-epithelialization was expected. Wound healing was photodocumented and evaluated using the Hollander Wound Evaluation Scale (HWES). Pain scores were evaluated daily according to the Visual Analogue Scale (VAS: from 1 to 10) and pain medication used by patients was recorded.

Results: Patients with Biatain Ibu dressing ($p<0.001$) and Suprathel ($p<0.004$) showed a statistically significant pain reduction up to two weeks postoperatively. No statistically significant difference was observed in re-epithelialization time, ease of use and patients satisfaction between the foam dressings and Suprathel. Six patients (three each with Mepilex Ag and with Suprathel) required extra pain medication.

Conclusions: The results of this study indicate that Biatain Ibu should be used as a standard dressing in elderly patients to reduce postoperative pain effectively. Suprathel fulfills the same qualities, but is more expensive. No statistically significant difference in handling and patient comfort, as well as patient satisfaction, was observed in the study.

ZUSAMMENFASSUNG

Hauttransplantation ist eine etablierte und häufig angewendete Methode um nicht oder schwer heilende Wunden oder Verbrennungen mit Haut oder Hautersatz zu decken. Verbände von Wunden solcher Art sind nach wie vor eine Herausforderung, um optimale Ergebnisse zu erzielen. Die Spalthautentnahmestellen sind nicht selten schmerzvoller als die Wunden, die mit den Hautteilen gedeckt werden. Aufgrund dieser zusätzlichen Wundfläche sind diese PatientInnen schmerzsensibler und bedürfen wegen des erhöhten Alters und eventueller Komorbidität besonderer Aufmerksamkeit.

Das Ziel dieser Studie war es, drei verschiedene hochqualifizierte Verbandsstoffe für Spalthautentnahmestellen an älteren PatientInnen (ab 55 Jahren) in einer prospektiven klinischen Studie zu testen. Die Spalthaut wurde nach standardisierter Methode geerntet und die Entnahmestellen unter sterilen Kautelen mit Biatain Ibu, Mepilex Ag oder Suprathel verbunden. Anhand der Visuellen Analogue Scale (VAS) wurden täglich Schmerzwerte erhoben und zusätzliche Schmerzmedikation notiert. Nach 10 bis 14 Tagen - nach zu erwartender Reepithelialisierug - wurde der Verband abgenommen, der Abheilungsgrad nach der Hollander Wound Evaluation Scale (HWES) bewertet und die Wunde/Narbe fotografiert. Anhand von Fragebögen wurden Handhabung und Effizienz der Verbände als auch die Patientenzufriedenheit erfasst.

Biatain Ibu (p<0.001) und Suprathel (p<0.004) zeigten innerhalb dieser 14 postoperativen Tage eine signifikante Schmerzreduktion. Bei Reepithelialisierung, Handhabung und Patientenzufriedenheit gab es keine nennenswerten Unterschiede zwischen allen drei Verbänden. Sechs PatientInnen (je drei Patienten mit Mepilex Ag und mit Suprathel) verlangten nach zusätzlichem Schmerzmittel.

Nachdem Schmerz eine nicht unwesentliche Bedeutung für die Wundheilung im Allgemeinen und bei älteren komorbiden PatientInnen im Besonderen hat, ist Biatain Ibu für diese Art der Wundheilung den anderen Verbänden zu bevorzugen. Handhabung und Patientenzufriedenheit sind sowohl bei beiden Schaumstoffverbänden als auch bei Suprathel ohne Unterschied. Bei annähernd gleicher Qualität sind die Schaumverbände kostenfreundlicher.

A prospective clinical trial comparing three different dressing materials for donor site wounds in elderly patients undergoing split-thickness skin graft surgery

INTRODUCTION

Transplantation medicine is one of the most challenging fields of modern medicine, forming an increasingly important aspect of regenerative medicine. Skin grafting, as a type of graft surgery, is a well-established surgical procedure that uses skin or a skin substitute to cover non-healing wounds or burns. This method was established and performed for thousands of years by surgeons to permanently replace damaged or missing skin. The progress of modern medicine has enabled the aging of patients suffering from chronic diseases like diabetes and hypertension, resulting in an increased number of patients in need of skin-grafting therapy due to diabetic ulcers, chronic wounds, burns or tumor wounds. Split-thickness graft therapy is an optimal way for patients to cover large or non-healing wounds with the body's own tissue (1). In addition to the actual wound grafting it requires the creation of a new wound at the donor site - which needs the best possible care to minimize infection and pain for the patients and to achieve optimal healing results (2, 3) especially in the elderly patient cohort. To achieve this aim, the choice of the dressing material used at the donor site wound is crucial (3). As new dressing products enter the market, there is an urgent need to evaluate which type of dressing to choose in order to fulfill the aforementioned needs for the donor site area (4).

1. THE SKIN

The character of skin varies greatly among individuals and its composition depends on the area of the body, genetic disposition, age, living circumstances and sun exposure. Skin consistency and texture change during a lifetime. In newborns and children, the skin is thin; from age 10 to 35 it thickens progressively and within the fourth decade, the skin thickness starts to decrease gradually until death. This decrease is attended by loss of skin elasticity and a progressive loss of sebaceous gland content (1).

The integument - the skin and its appendages - is the largest organ of the human body with several major functions including protection, thermoregulation, sensation, excretion and absorption (5). It fulfills the function of immunology, detoxication and retention and has a remarkable regenerative capacity. The skin interacts with the inside of the body and with our environment (6). Skin thickness ranges between 0.5 mm and 3 mm, and varies greatly with the body area. It is thinner on the face, neck and upper extremities; the skin of the eyelids is thinnest, while the skin is thickest on the back, the palms of the hands and soles of the feet and on the scalp (7).

The skin consists of two major layers, the epidermis (outer layer) and the dermis (inner layer) (8). The hypodermis consists of loose connective and adipose tissue (panniculus) affiliating the skin with its underlying structures, binding it via the superficious body fascia to the particular regions of the body (6) (Fig. 1). About 95% of the skin is dermis, and the residual 5% is epidermis (9, 10).

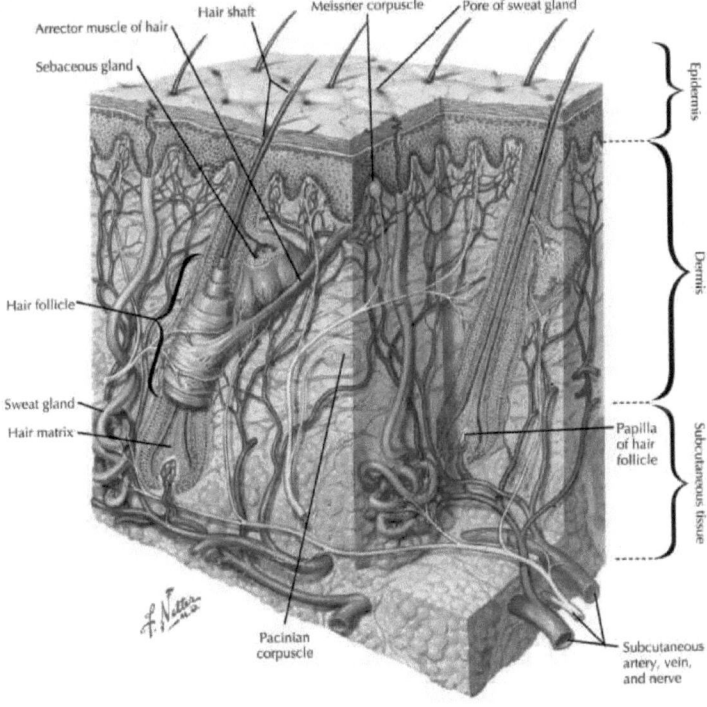

Figure 1. Schematic of skin and its appendages, epidermis, dermis and subcutaneous skin (Netter's Essential Histology, 2nd Edition, p.244) (10)

1.1 The Epidermis

The epidermis is 0.05 to 0.1mm thick and consists of a layer of keratinocytes and several layers of rapidly dividing cells underneath. More than 90% of the cell population of the epidermis is keratinocytes that provide protection and produce keratin, a complex filamentous protein. Other epidermal cells are Melanocytes (melanin producing cells in the bottom of the stratum basale), Merkel cells (slow adapting touch cells), which derive from the neural crest and Langerhans cells, which are important for immune defense. The epidermis is vascularized and innervated via the dermis by unencapsulated free nerve endings losing their myelin-sheaths when they enter the epidermis (10). The color of the skin depends on the melanin produced (6). There is a permanent renewal of this outer layer, consisting of five different sheets - stratum corneum, stratum lucidum, stratum granulosum, stratum spinosum and stratum basale (Fig. 2 and Fig. 3), where cells from bottom to the top undergo mitosis, differentiation, maturation and are finally shed from the skin after keratinization (9). Slow cycling stem cells provide a reservoir for regeneration of the epidermis. Stem cells divide infrequently in normal skin, but in cell culture they form active growing colonies (11). The basement membrane forms the border to the dermis and describes a matrix layer from which all of its cells originate (10).

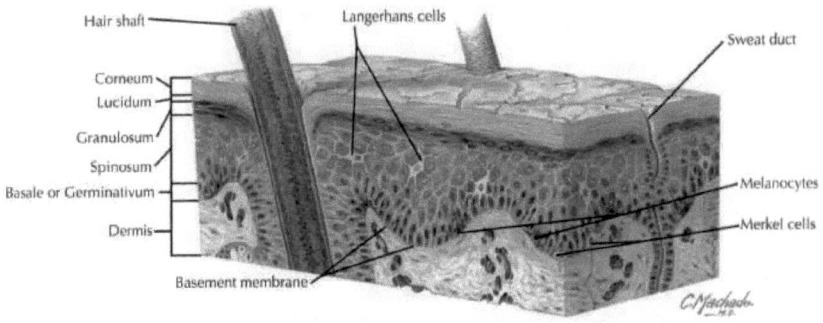

Figure 2. Strata of epidermis (Netter's Essential Histology, 2nd Edition, p.246) (10)

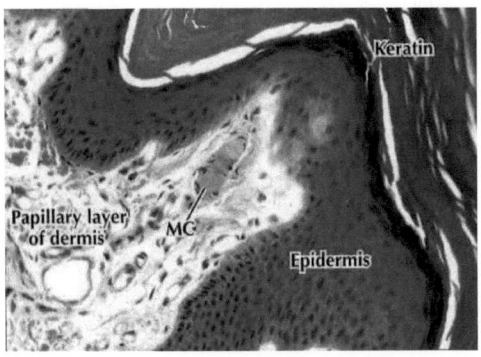

Figure 3. Light micrograph of thick skin at the dermoepidermal junction; MC: Meissner corpuscle = tactile corpuscle (Netter's Essential Histology, 2nd Edition, p.246) (10)

1.2 The Dermis

The dermis (corium) is the fundament of the skin (6) and consists of two parts, the external papillar layer and the internal reticular layer. The papillar dermis represents the sensory part of the skin, where inflammatory reactions occur (9). The reticular dermis has few cells, containing an extensive meshed network mainly from type I collagen accompanied by thick elastic fibrills which give the skin reversibility, dilatability and tear strength. Collagen, the major structural protein for the entire body, represents 70% of the dry weight of the skin, of which the fibrillar collagen represents the major group (12).

The dermis is richly vascularized by large muscular arteries and veins that are found in the subcutaneous connective tissue. The deeper reticular plexus and a more superficial papillary plexus are connected together (Fig. 4 and Fig. 5). The dermis also contains sebaceous glands, sweat glands close to the connecting tissue and hair follicles (10). There exists a complex network of sensory nerves and efferent sympathetic innervation of sweat glands and arrector pili muscles (smooth muscles) throughout the dermis (9).

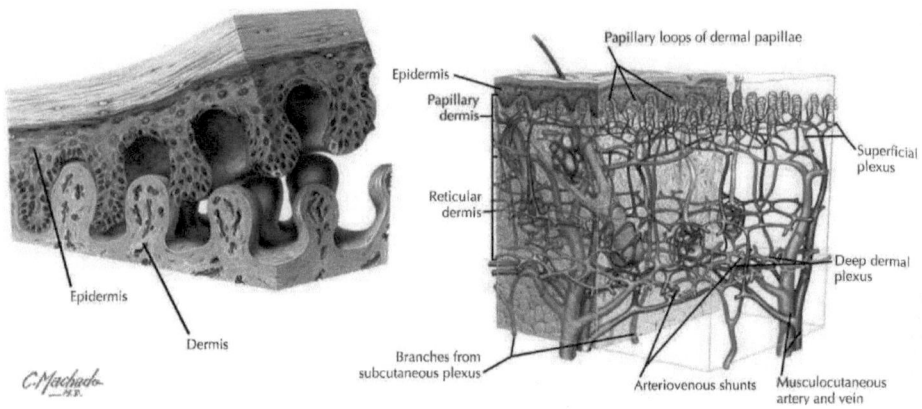

Figure 4. Blood supply to dermis (Netters Essential Histology, 2nd Edition, p. 252) (10)

The skin appendages are mainly of epithelial origin. They arise from the deflection in the epidermis and are formed under regulatory influence of the dermis. Hence, they require a live interaction between the dermis and the epidermis (10). While the various adnexal structures serve specific functions, they all can act as reserve epidermis in the re-epithelialization after injury by the migration of keratinocytes from the adnexal epithelium to the skin surface (9).

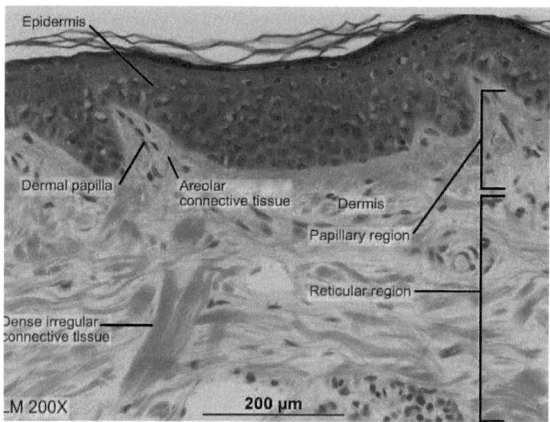

Figure 5. Light micrograph of skin layers, epidermis, papillary and reticular dermis (13)

12

1.3 The Subcutaneous Tissue

The subcutaneous tissue consists of a meshwork of connective tissue with lobes of fat inside. They reach the stratum reticulare of the dermis, as well as the straight connective tissue of the firm underlying structures like muscles, tendons or bone, where they fix as so-called "retinacula cutis", the skin with the deeper body structures. This is important for sensory receptor-communication and balancing pressure, mainly on the palms of the hands and the soles of the feet (9).

2. SKIN GRAFTING

Skin grafting is a well-established surgical procedure (14), successfully used   for over a century to cover superficial defects of any kind in the skin (7). The transplanted skin closes and protects the wound bed against trauma and infection and helps to regain functionality and the aesthetic look, which is of utmost importance for all patients.

2.1 General Aspects

A skin graft consists of epidermis and the dermis (parts of it or the whole) depending on the graft type chosen (15). Grafts of any kind, including skin grafts, require and depend on vascularization, which is crucial for their survival.

Various types of grafts have been described. In an autograft procedure undamaged skin from another part of the patient's own body is transformed to cover a skin defect in a different part of the body of the same individual. An iso- or syngraft is a graft between genetically identical individuals of the same species.
An allograft is taken from another individual of the same species. A xenograft (heterograft) is a graft, taken from an individual of one species grafted onto an individual of a different species (7).

2.2 Historical Background

Free skin grafts had already been used as early as 2500 to 3000 BC in India (16). Called the "Ancient Indian Method", they used free grafts of skin, including subcutaneous fat that they took from the gluteal region, mainly to reconstruct ears and noses, which had been severed as punishment. The Indian surgeon Sushruta (600 BC) is called the "father of plastic surgery" for his description of the reconstruction of earlobes and rhinoplasty for a severed nose in the "Sushruta samita", which is still valid today. The operation, where a new nose was reconstructed with skin of the forehead in several steps, was reserved to the members of the brickmakers' cast (17).

From the beginning of the first millennium until the Middle Ages, knowledge about the survival of tissue was small. The earliest attempts of grafting were undertaken to replace amputated parts of the body. At the beginning of the 16th century, surgeons began to study the effects of removing and replacing pieces of skin on animals trying to reconstruct noses with free skin flaps from the arm (17). Ambroise Paré (1510-1590), a French surgeon, as well as the Italian surgeon Gaspare Tagliacozzi (1546-1599), known as one of the pioneers of plastic surgery for describing exact reconstruction techniques for the nose, ear and lip, contributed considerably to establish plastic surgery as it is known today (18).

Giuseppe Baronio (1759-1811), an Italian physiologist, performed the first professional medical experiments with skin grafts in a series of animals, where he transferred various thicknesses of skin of various sizes at variable times. All the grafts were successful and started bleeding when cut off again. His findings are carefully recorded in "Degli Innesti Animali" of 1804 (19).

Christian Heinrich Bunger (1782-1842), a German anatomist and surgeon, reported the partly successful transplantation of a free whole-thickness skin graft for the repair of a nasal defect in 1823. Sir Astley Cooper (1768-1841), an English surgeon and anatomist, was the first to remove skin from an amputated thumb to cover the stump. In 1869, the Swiss surgeon Jean-Louis Reverdin (1842-1929) detached bits of transplanted skin cut out with a scissor, to observe the healing of granulating wounds. He took thin parts of the epidermis only and called them "epidermic grafts", now known as "pinch grafts", small islands from which the epithelium spreads out from the individual islands that are grafted (20). These grafts contained a portion of dermis, as Reverdin later admitted.

In 1872, the French orthopedic surgeon Louis Ollier (1830-1900) developed a split-thickness skin graft modified later by the German surgeon Carl Thiersch (1822–1895) in 1886 (21). Thus the names Ollier and Thiersch are synonymous today with thin (0.005-0.001 inch = 0.13-0.25 mm) split-thickness grafts. Later the Ollier-Thiersch type of graft became much thicker and was called the "split-graft" (Blair and Brown). They also recognized that the depth of the graft is an important factor in donor site healing.

Lawson (1870), Le Fort (1872) and Wolfe (1876) used full-thickness grafts for ectropion therapy of the lower eyelid. Wolfe and Krause were mainly involved in the improvement of this method, known today as "Wolfe-Krause grafts" (22).
In 1942, Brown and McDowell reported using thick split-thickness grafts (0.01-0.022 inch = 0.25-0.56 mm) for the treatment of burns (23). This was improved by Tanner,

14

Vandeput, and Olley in 1964 (24), when they expanded skin grafts with a machine up to 12 times their original surface area.

Ten years later, epithelial skin culture technology started with Rheinwald and Green in 1975 (25). Rudolph and coworkers reported in 1976 that the dermal component of grafted skin exerts an important influence on wound contraction (26, 27). The first human keratinocytes were grown from an epithelial layer in 1979 which marked the beginning of the era of tissue engineering (27, 28).

Techniques of harvesting split-thickness skin grafts changed over time. Long cutting blades were replaced by the mechanical dermatome, which was replaced by the electrodermatome being used today. This device enables plastic surgeons to harvest skin grafts with a thickness from 0.30 to 0.50 mm (Fig. 6).

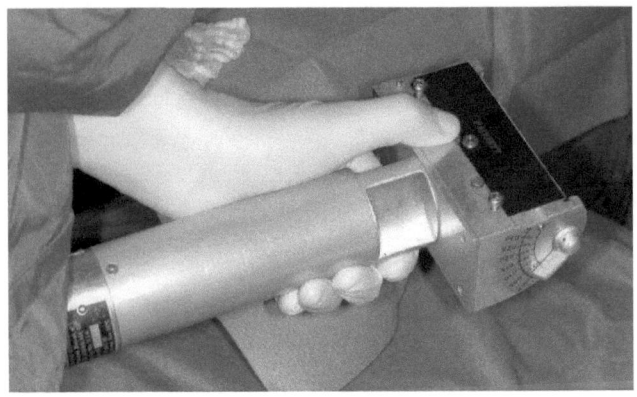

Figure 6. Modern electrodermatome (Department of Plastic Surgery, LKH Graz)

2.3 Skin Graft Types

Skin grafts are classified as partial or split-thickness skin graft (STSG) and full-thickness skin graft (FTSG), depending on how much of the dermis is harvested. All skin grafts must include at least a portion of dermal layer for survival. The graft interferes with the transport of nutrients to the important upper skin layers. Therefore, no fat should be included in the skin graft (15).

<u>Full-Thickness Skin Graft (FTSG)</u>

A full thickness skin graft (FTSG) consists of two main layers of the skin (epidermis and dermis) and needs a well-vascularized recipient bed. It is mainly used to cover facial wounds for aesthetic reasons, or wounds where there is a strong mechanical demand – like on the palms or soles. Because of the unavailable regeneration of the wound bed, full thickness skin grafts are limited. The wound on the donor site has to be closed by suture (15). FTSGs contract less upon healing, they show better trauma-resistance and they have a more natural look when healed (7).

<u>Split-Thickness Skin Graft (STSG)</u>

Split-thickness grafts (STSG) contain the epidermis and varying amounts of the dermis (Fig.7). As the deep dermis (reticular dermis) in the donor site area is spared by the surgeon, it enables the wound bed to regenerate itself. Skin grafts can be harvested from every part of the body, but typical donor site areas include the buttock, thigh, back, or abdominal wall, sites that are normally hidden by clothes of the patients. The skin is harvested mainly from the thigh that is well supplied with blood and is not too close to the bones which improves the aesthetic appearance of the donor site. The graft is harvested by using an electrodermatome (Fig. 6) which is applied to the donor site area (7). Thin split-thickness skin grafts have the best "take" but as a disadvantage they tend to shrink, to pigment abnormally and they are prone to trauma (26).

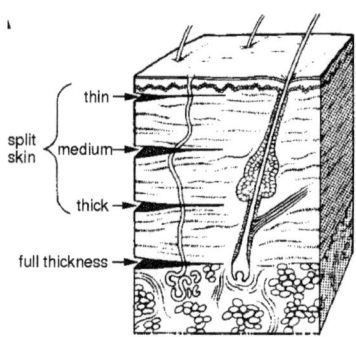

Figure 7. Skin graft types (Grabb & Smith's Plastic Surgery, 6th Edition, p. 8) (15)

A graft can be laid in the form of a sheet (sheet skin graft) with the advantage of a continuous uninterrupted surface and a better aesthetic outcome. The disadvantage

16

of this graft type lies in not allowing fluid to pass through, thus complicating healing (15).

Meshed grafts are sheet grafts with multiple mechanical incisions (Fig. 10) to enlarge the sheet by one-half or more to gain multiple extensions to cover large wounds. The incisions allow fluid to pass through into the dressing thereby preventing the formation of hematomas or seromas on the recipient site. This technique spares the patient a large donor site wound, but results in a reticulated appearance at the recipient wound site after healing (29).

Micrograft Techniques

Pinch/Punch Graft

Almost one hundred years ago, John Staige Davis (21) used a modified version of Reverdin's method of creating skin grafts which became known as the "pinch graft". The pinch graft is a small rounded deep graft (3 to 5 mm in diameter) containing all the layers of the skin. A needle is used to pick up a cone of skin, which - after cutting it at its base with a knife - is brought to the recipient wound bed. One avoids to place the skin island to close in wound area in order to allow a free discharge (25). If the skin is cut as a plug with a biopsy punch, it is called a punch graft.

This type of skin grafting is used for granulating wounds, small wounds on the limbs, wounds with low-grade infection or contaminated wounds. They are predominantly used to promote epithelialization from the wound edge as well as from the skin islands. Nowadays, the pinch-graft has been widely replaced by attentive excision of the skin bed and coverage by split-thickness skin graft, as has been the punch graft method by the invention of dermatomes to produce mesh skin grafts (29).

Patch graft

The patch graft technique was first reported by Gabarro in 1943 (22). It was accomplished by removing a donor piece of skin of a certain size (one-sixth to one ninth of the wound size), which was placed on a piece of paper, then cut into small squares, and then placed onto the wound bed. This method has been almost entirely replaced by the advent of dermatomes (30, 31).

Meek Microdermagraft

This technique is named after C. Parker Meek (32), who harvested a thin split-thickness graft and placed it on a cork carrier with the dermal side down. This cork carrier is then placed on a cutting block of a microdermatome to create microskin grafts. This technique (33) was developed for the re-epithelialization of small skin pieces where the wound area is quite large and requires the largest possible number of growing margins (29).

Chinese Intermingled Technique

This technique was developed in China in the 1980s and combines skin autografts and allografts for covering large burn wounds (31). When donor sites for autologous skin were limited (30, 31), a sheet of allograft is wrapped around the wound, and holes are punched out about 1 cm apart on the allograft skin. The holes are "filled" with autograft skin from the scalp. When the autograft skin migrates in between the allograft's dermis and epidermis this is called the "sandwich phenomenon" (31).

Microskin Graft

With growing interest in this field and greater advancements of scientific research, a new technique with some patch grafting and an intermingled technique was generated. This technique involves a small piece of autograft skin being minced with scissors into small pieces (< 1mm^3), then brought into saline, where the skin parts are able to direct themselves with the epidermis upward (34). The small pieces of skin are dispersed on a silk cloth, overlaid by a sheet of split-thickness allograft and then transferred as the graft to the wound.

Many more micrograft-techniques exist, and/or modified or taken in combination with those mentioned above. They are used especially in patients with burn injuries (29), and are parallel developments to the very active research in the field of artificial skin (35).

2.4 Modern Skin Grafts – The Surgical Procedure

Before being able to place and suture the graft to the recipient area, the surgeon will undertake a proper and careful preparation of the wound, as skin grafts do not usually survive on tissue with limited blood supply. The wound has to be cleaned of necrotic tissue particles by debridement; foreign material or any bacterial contamination has to be removed. The wound will then be rinsed with saline or mild antiseptics. To enable proper suturing, epinephrine can be applied on the wound to constrict blood vessels. Graft placement can even sometimes be delayed when the wound bed is too infected (30).

The skin graft must be held in proximity to the wound bed, which is achieved by suturing the graft in place and using a firm dressing to avoid shearing. Tie-over packs will be necessary in cases where small skin grafts have to be secured (neck or head area) or where deep defects (axilla wounds) have to be covered (15).

A skin graft harvested from the donor site is completely separated from its blood supply. Brought to its new position, the graft initially survives by diffusion of nutrients from the wound bed into the graft. This keeps the graft alive for the first 3 to 5 days and is called imbibition. After 48 hours, an anastomosis between recipient vessels and vessels in the skin graft starts to set in. This step is called inosculation, followed by revascularization and replacement of the fibrin network which first acts as a biological glue and adheres the graft to the wound bed (36). By infiltration with fibroblasts a fibrous tissue attachment is formed. Blood vessels in the wound bed start to form endothelial buds and meet the blood vessels in the skin graft which gives the graft a red-purple color (26, 36). A physiological integration of the skin graft into the recipient site is called "take" (37). Maturing of the graft continues by regaining partial sensation from the sensory nerves of the wound bed (38).

The following figures (Fig. 8 to Fig. 10, Photographs taken at the Department of Plastic Surgery, LKH Graz) demonstrate the harvest of a split-thickness skin graft; Figure 10 shows how it is enlarged by meshing.

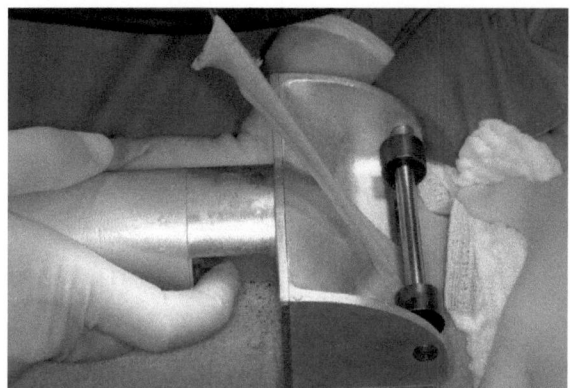

Figure 8. First slide of harvest

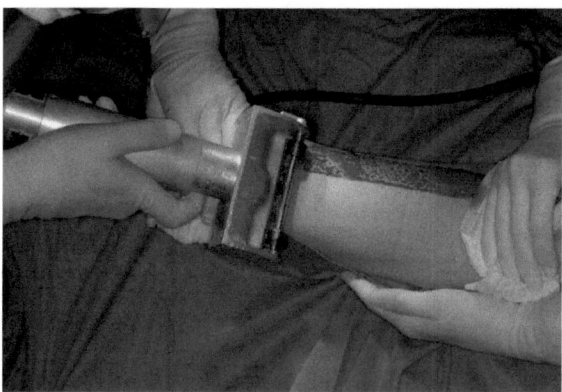

Figure 9. Beginning of second slide harvest. It is important to keep the skin taut and to apply appropriate pressure while operating the electrodermatome.

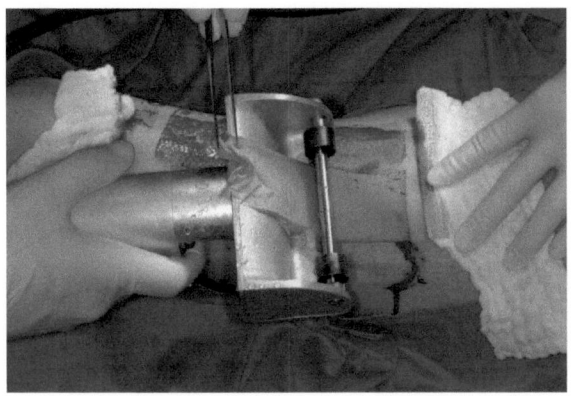

Figure 10. Second slide harvest. The skin sheet is thin and must be handled with care; it is placed in saline before being meshed.

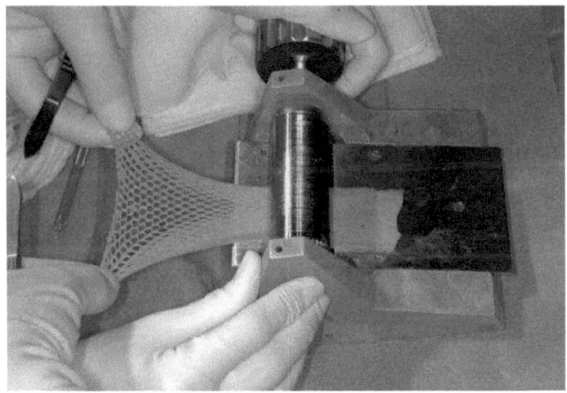

Figure 11. Transformation of a sheet skin graft into a meshed graft to increase volume and to allow wound drainage.

2.5 Postoperative Aspects of Skin Grafts and Donor Sites

The donor site regenerates by re-epithelialization. Epidermal cells immigrate from the hair follicle shafts and adnexal structures of the dermis. This regeneration capacity is specific to the epidermis and is not existent in the dermis. Therefore, the number of split-thickness skin grafts from one particular part of the body is dependent on the thickness of the donor dermis (15).

All skin grafts contract immediately after removal from the donor site. The more dermis the graft contains, the more contraction will be experienced. The secondary contracture happens later at the donor site as a result of the activity of myofibroblasts. It depends on the thickness of the skin graft: the thinner the graft, the greater the secondary contracture. Full thickness skin grafts contract more on initial harvest.

Skin grafts are reinnervated by ingrowth of nerve fibers from the place to which they are transplanted. It depends on the portion of dermis harvested, as well as on how much of the epithelial appendages are transferred. The greatest sensory return is achieved by full thickness skin grafts, because of a greater availability of nerve sheaths (15).

In general, full thickness skin grafts produce the hair growth of the donor site, whereas split-thickness skin grafts, especially thin thickness skin grafts - depending on the dermis portion - are generally hairless. After re-epithelialization, the scar should constantly be nourished with oil-based ointment to prevent it from drying out. Similarly to every other scar, it should be protected against sun for one year to minimize scarring. Donor sites are deep red during the first months (Fig.19) and become pale within one year, until they appear only slightly lighter than the surrounding skin (30). They regain all the missing properties back, including functionality, and theoretically can be donor sites again.

Donor sites may be extremely painful and vulnerable for infection. Careful preparation and meticulous inspection of the graft can minimize infection and the risk of loss. Causes of graft failure can be bleeding or serum collection beneath the graft, which disrupts proper nutrition. Further risks in split-thickness skin grafting can be infection or nerve damage.

2.6 Wound Healing

Any injury to the skin integrity is potentially harmful as it will disrupt the functions noted above and will cause pain to the patient. Depending on the size, depth and localization, a wound will either heal by itself with little or no scarring or it must be sutured by a physician. When wounds are extensive, closure by suturing will not be possible and skin grafting is necessary to cover the wound and minimize scarring.

By definition, wound healing might include the repair or reconstitution of a defect in an organ or tissue, mainly in the skin (15). This requires a complex process that is best demonstrated in cutaneous wound healing. The intrinsic and extrinsic clotting systems are activated and acute and chronic inflammatory responses start to happen (Fig.12). Neovascularization begins, furthermore cell proliferation, division, apoptosis and migration are necessary to deposit the extracellular matrix and to remodel it (39).

Wound healing may occur in different ways according to time and efforts at treatment. Healing by primary intention (sanatio per primam intentionem, p.p.) mainly describes a wound closed by approximation of wound margins or by placement of a graft or a flap, and takes place in the case of wounds created in the operation room. It occurs directly without intervention of granulations, it heals with a scar and it does not require special wound care.

Wound healing by secondary intention (sanatio per secundam intentionem, p.s.) occurs when wounds are left open to prevent infection and the subsequent defect is filled with granulation tissue and then re-epithelialized. For these wounds, special wound care and treatments are necessary. When wounds are highly contaminated, and only delayed closure is possible, it is called healing by third intention.

Acute wounds are those for which injury has occurred up to a month previously. If wounds are persisting beyond 4 to 6 weeks or longer, these wounds are considered chronic wounds, as are wounds that do not heal for months or years (40).

2.6.1 Wound management from ancient history to modern times

Wound care management is an important cornerstone of modern medicine. The first steps in treatment of wounds were already taken in ancient history as it was realized that hygiene was a key factor to ensure proper wound healing. The history of surgery has been the history of wound therapy since the beginning of mankind.

Wounds are associated with pain, hemorrhage and loss of skin continuity and tissue substances (41). Attempts to handle wound care were always an experiment in trial and error. Medical knowledge has evolved in every highly developed culture. Some of these cultures had primitive methods, while others had some highly developed healing methods. The first written records date from about 2500 BC from Mesopotamia, where wounds were washed with water or milk and were dressed with honey, resin, or myrrh. The useful effect of many plants has been used for healing over thousands of years and continues to be used today. Bandages could have been made of linen or wool (42).

In the Ebers Papyrus, dated to ca 1550 BC (after Georg Ebers, a German Egyptologist), the Egyptians described the use of linseed and honey in wound management. They also introduced many minerals into wound treatment and already observed that closed wounds heal better than open ones. In order to incorporate this knowledge, they invented the adhesive bandage to draw wound edges together. Massive bleeding may have been treated with cauterisation (43).

Greek medicine was influenced by the Egyptians. The Greek medical tradition began with Asklepios, the god of medicine and healing in ancient Greek religion (41). The first Greek medical references were found in Homer's Iliad (800 BC). Hippocrates of Kos (460-377 BC), an ancient Greek physician, is known as one of the most important figures in the history of medicine. He suggested that contused wounds should be treated with salves in order to promote suppuration, remove necrotic material and reduce inflammation. Hippokrates differentiated between ordinary wounds without detritus and complicated wounds, and he advocated that the majority of wounds should be kept dry. It was common to clean wounds with wine or vinegar and cover them with a fat or oil-based balm (44).

Aulus Cornelius Celsus (25 BC-50 AD) was considered one of the most important contributors to medicine and science during the Roman Empire - he was the first to mention the four characteristics of inflammation (rubor, calor, tumor, donor) that later were rediscovered by Rudolf Virchow (1821-1902), a German pathologist (39). Celsus differentiated between wounds and chronic sores and also mentioned that they required different management. He advocated the primary suture of fresh wounds and the debridement of contused or contaminated wounds to convert them back to fresh wounds that could then be sutured. The fifth characteristic of inflammation (functio laesa) was added by Galenos of Pergamon (129-216 AD), famous for his four element theory (fire, earth, air and water). Even as early as the third century he acknowledged the importance of maintaining wound site moisture to ensure successful closure of the wound. He brought medical knowledge from the Orient to the Arabs. By the end of the tenth century the dominant centre of Islamic medicine had come from Bagdad to Cordoba. Thus, early European surgery was influenced by Galenos. Islamic medicine made a number of important scientific contributions including the discovery of distillation and crystallization – and Arab knowledge in chemistry provided the first scientific base of pharmacy. The first European medical school was founded at Salerno in the ninth century (41).

Most milestones in wound treatment were reached mainly during the 19th century and the beginning of the 20th century. The introduction of antiseptic in surgery played an important role. Joseph Lister (1827-1912), an English surgeon, inspired by applying the work of the French chemist Louis Pasteur (1822-1895) - the "father of microbiology" and an advocate of the germ theory of disease, based on the works of Fracastoro, Bassi and Henle (45) introduced antiseptic in surgery by sterilizing instruments. He discovered that carbolic acid that was swabbed on wounds remarkably reduced the incidence of gangrene. Instruments were washed in the same solution and assistants sprayed the solution in the operating theatre.

Ignaz Semmelweis (1818-1865), an Austro-Hungarian physician, reduced the mortality rate of women dying of puerperal fever (childbed fever) enormously, when he gave advice to his doctors to clean their hands with chlorinated lime solution when changing from the section room to the obstetrical clinic. He knew only about the existence of cadaveric pathogens, but did not understand exactly what they were.

This was discovered in the same century by many famous physicians and scientists who made essential achievements in modern medicine and natural sciences. Representative of these are Robert Koch (1843-1910), a German physician, who together with Ferdinand J. Cohn (1828-1898), a German plant pathologist, is considered one of the founders of bacteriology, as well as Sir Alexander Fleming (1881-1955), a Scottish bacteriologist, widely regarded for his discovery of penicillin in 1928 (45).

2.6.2 Modern standards in wound management

The concept of moist wound healing (MWH) is relatively new. It was first supported by John Bull et al in 1948 (46), and later demonstrated by George Winter in 1962 (47), and Howard Maibach (Hinman and Maibach 1963) by experimental studies on animals (domestic pigs) where they could show that epithelialization occurred twice as fast when wounds were kept moist. Until this finding, the interim view was to allow wounds to dry out and promote healing by forming scabs (40, 41).
A scab or eschar is the endpoint of drying out a wound and consists of the epidermis and the superficial dermis (48). The results have been taken as representative of all wound healing situations and MWH is a basic principle of modern wound management (49).

"Moist wound healing" is not clearly defined and is sometimes described as "not too wet, not too dry" (49). It advocates that the optimal environment for the repair and restoration of tissue function is one in which the wound bed is kept moist for providing an ideal context in which the essential components of natural wound healing as described below can develop (50). Physiologically, the body provides a moist wound environment by producing exudate, which under exposure to the atmosphere transforms into a scab, covering the re-epithelialization of the wound bed with a physiological barrier and repelled as eschar (43, 44).
A moist wound environment permits the possibility of increasing macrophage and fibroblast activity, re-epithelialization and collagen production. Moisture is important for cell movement and the gene-expression which is needed for repair activity (51).

Consequently, moist wound healing is the basic principle of wound treatment today and a standard for current dressing materials and methods (52).

2.6.3 Steps of wound healing

Normal wound healing in mammals occurs in four overlapping but distinct biological phases: coagulation, the inflammatory phase, the proliferative phase and epithelialization and remodeling phase (Fig.12), which is completed by scar formation.

Coagulation

Immediately after tissue injury, the wound healing process is initiated by platelets releasing mediators, including platelet-derived growth factor (PDGF), insulin-like growth factor-1 (IGF-1), epidermal growth factor (EGF), and fibroblast growth factor (FGF). First, hemostasis is stimulated by components of the injured tissue. Devitalized tissue is removed by phagocytosis by macrophages to prevent infection by microbial pathogens. Bleeding is stopped by activation of the clotting cascade. Finally, fibrinogen is converted to fibrin, and following polymerization, a mesh is formed. Growth factors work as mitogens to stimulate proliferation of wound cells; some are stimulating migration of target cells (chemotaxis) and have regulating potential (53).

The Inflammatory Phase

The inflammatory phase is named and characterized by inflammatory cells that are attracted by numerous biophysical cues, initiating the steps of the complement cascade. It is initiated by the blood clotting and platelet degranulation process and shows vasodilation, increased capillary permeability, complement activation and migration of polymorph nuclear endocytes and macrophages. Damaged ECM is degraded by elastase and collagenase which secrete new growth factors like TGF-b, TGF-a, heparin-binding epidermal growth factor (HB-EGF) and basic fibroblast growth factor (bFGF) (53). The wound cavity caused by injury, is filled with neutrophils and prepared for healing by committed progenitor and mature cells of hematopoiesis. After 48 hours, circulating monocytes follow neutrophils into the wound, which happens up to 72 hours post-injury. They traffic the wound and transform to macrophages. After 3 days, they are the predominant cell type in the healing wound. The last cell to enter the wound is the lymphocyte, 5 to 7 days post-wounding.

The Proliferative Phase

The proliferative phase of wound healing consists of re-epithelialization and may last from day 4 to day 21 after injury. Re-epithelialization probably begins shortly after injury and means tissue-replacement with the same structure and function as before. Otherwise it is called reparation, and means to replace destroyed parenchymal cells with collagen connective tissue (39). In this phase, the desmosomal connections and the underlying basement membrane become loose, so that cells from the basement membrane are freed and begin to migrate laterally. The fibrin matrix, formed in the first phase of wound repair is replaced by a new migration-platform, the granulation tissue. This tissue is characterized by three cell types: fibroblasts, macrophages and endothelial cells. Endothelial cells are a critical component of granulation tissue - they are able to form new blood vessels, to induce angiogenesis and vasculogenesis (15). Extracellular matrix (ECM) is produced by fibroblasts and fills the healing scar. Macrophages, producing growth factors such as PDGF and TGF-ß-1, enable fibroblasts to proliferate and migrate and stimulate endothelial cells to form new vessels. The provisional fibrin-mesh is replaced with thinner type III collagen, which later will be replaced by the more powerful type I collagen (both fibrillated collagens and therefore structure proteins) as it was before (10).

The Remodeling Phase

The final phase is the remodeling phase. It describes the longest episode of wound healing and lasts from day 2 up to 1 year or longer. This phase starts after granulation and keratinocyte migration and re-epithelialization with regression of blood vessels. After collagen replacement the wound is contracted by myofibroblasts that later disappear. The migration-process, already induced from the basement cellular layer, starts from the edges of the wound where the epidermis newly starts to differentiate (39).

Skin sites such as the face or scalp, which contain a lot of pilosebaceous units, re-epithelialize more rapidly than do skin sites where adnexa of all types are sparsely found, such as the back. Once a wound has re-epithelialized, granulation tissue is no longer produced. Therefore, wounds in an area with few adnexa will slowly fill with granulation tissue. In contrast, areas with numerous adnexa will quickly be covered with epithelium (12). The response to injury always depends on the wounded tissue, on the diseases, and on environmental factors, as well as on the individual (54).

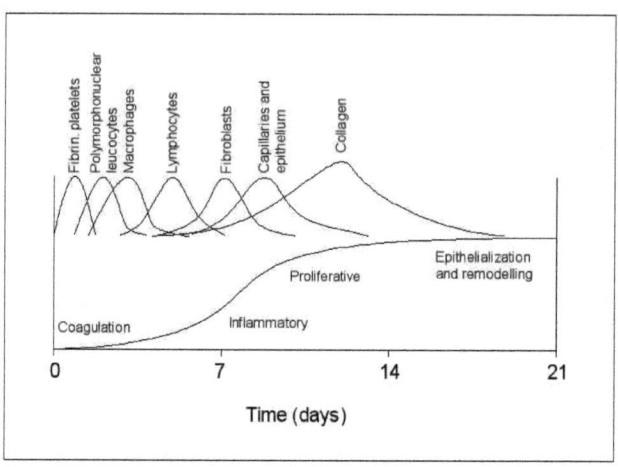

Figure 12. Wound healing phases (53)

Scar Formation

According to Ferguson a scar in the skin may be defined as "a macroscopic disturbance of the normal structure and function of the skin architecture resulting of the end product of a healed wound". Thus, skin scars are the biological outcome of mammalian tissue repair. A temporary cellular matrix rebuilds the continuity of the wound before a reactivation for re-creation of the missing tissue is started. During normal wound healing, myofibroblasts finally disappear after the re-epithelialization process as described previously. The theory of evolution advocates that wounds heal quickly to prevent infection, and scars are the best price humankind pays for survival.

Scar formation depends on individual and genetic (age, sex, race) background, on tissue site and on body location (55). Scarless skin healing only occurs in early mammalian embryos and invertebrates (56). The more pigmented the skin, the more scarring. In children and adolescents, scarring is severe because of an increased turnover of the cells. The skin of the shoulders and the breastbone tends to form the worst scars, whereas intraoral tissue scars the least. Scars show a wide spectrum of clinical phenotypes: from fine, pale lines, to hypertrophic or hypotrophic scars, elevated or nodular scars, ranging also to contractures or keloids with aesthetic and functional limitation (57).

2.6.4 Wound management of the donor recipient graft site

Due to exposure of sensory nerve endings (58), the donor site wound is often more painful than the skin graft wound. The healing process occurs through re-epithelialization by remnants in the reticular dermis. The duration of the wound healing process usually varies between 7 to 21 days (Fig. 12) depending on the age, general health condition and nutritional status of the patient.

Appropriate dressing for the donor site is vital to the patient as removal of a dressing can cause pain. Dressing materials have to fulfill the needs of the wound healing phases. Normally the donor site wound produces a lot of exudate in the first days (wet phase) when an absorbent dressing should be applied to absorb the excess fluid. When the wound bed starts to become dry (dry phase) after 3 to 4 days postoperatively, a non-adherent function of the dressing should be desirable so that it does not adhere to the wound bed which can remain undisturbed in situ for several days not disrupting the re-epithelialization process. In addition to the choice of the most suitable dressing, which should be in expert hands, optimal pain management should be offered to the patients (30).

2.6.5 Wound dressing

Wound dressings have existed for as long as there have been wounds. The use of linen soaked in oil or grease continued for at last 4000 years until woven absorbent cotton gauze was introduced in 1817 (41). The awareness of the impact of wound dressings was already mentioned in the Edwin Smith Surgical Papyrus, dating back to 1615 BC: "closed wounds heal more quickly than open wounds" (59). Also, the knowledge of antisepsis and microorganisms in the late 1800s had a great impact on this field (44). Until the mid-1900s, man believed that wounds healed more quickly if kept dry and uncovered. In 1948, Oscar Gilje described the "moist chamber effect" for healing ulcers (60) and in 1962, George Winter conducted a landmark study in his works on moist wound healing (47).

Historically, wound dressings simply provided protection to the wound surface. In modern times, a range of synthetic/semisynthetic or natural dressing materials are available that support or interact with the wound healing process in many ways.

To date, according to Morgan (61) and Thomas (62) the most essential requirements of the ideal wound dressing should guarantee the following attributes:

Essential Requirements

- be free of toxic or irritant components
- not release particles or non-biodegradable fibres into the wound
- form an effective bacterial barrier
- be self-adhesive and form a water-resistant seal to the surrounding skin
- produce minimal pain during application and removal
- provide an optimal state of hydration
- maintain optimum temperature and pH
- allow gaseous exchange

Additional Requirements

- antimicrobial activity
- hemostatic properties
- capability to remove or inactivate proteolytic enzymes in exudate
- release of pain medication
- wound cleansing activity
- odor-absorbing/neutralizing properties

Wounds can be dressed with biologic or with synthetic materials in open, semi-open and occlusive manners (7).

Occlusive wound dressings are utilized to accelerate wound healing and improve the final appearance of scars (63). Acute wounds that heal under occlusion show accelerated healing stages, a greater strength and a better cosmetic outcome (59). Semi-open wound dressings are characterized by the possibility of applying topical products or antiseptics and gauze bandages and allowing fluid drainage into the outer dressing. It ensures ventilation and thermal protection. One property of semi-occlusive dressings is oxygen exchange. Most commonly, multiple dressing changes are made until the wound is healed (64).

When wounds are left open, the healing duration is prolonged, and it is associated with more pain and higher risk of complication (7).

Otherwise, as described by Allen et al (65), wounds left open to granulate are more sterile than wounds covered with skin dressings. Although covered wounds showed microbial flora. Szabo et al found out, that skin grafts have no intrinsic bactericidal properties (66), a fact, that is replaced in some dressing materials, like Mepilex Ag.

Modern dressing started with the invention of fibrous synthetics such as nylon, polyethylene and polyvinyl. Later improvements were achieved in composite and hybrid polymers, which amplified the wound dressing material available and permanently expanded it with temporary skin substitutes and the innovative field of tissue engineering (67).

In particular, the dressing material used for the donor site must provide the optimum healing environment to allow the wound an undisturbed healing process, and so guarantee proper re-epithelialization. It should prevent infection and trauma, be comfortable for the patient, thus not causing any pain, assure easy handling and have a good correlation between cost and benefit (64).

The range of wound dressings can be subcategorized as follows:

Types of wound dressings
Low adherent dressings Semipermeable dressings Hydrogels and hydrocolloids Alginates Film Foam Composite dressings Antimicrobials Sprays Temporary artificial skin substitutes

Absorbent dressings have to be used if skin graft sites or donor sites produce large amounts of exudate. To prevent maceration of the skin graft and the surrounding skin, foam dressings, alginate or hydrofiber dressing should be preferred. Antimicrobial dressings, like silver dressing, can be necessary to reduce the bacterial load of the recipient site (50).

The following short description of the dressing types is taken out of "Wound Dressings", by Jones, Grey, Harding, 2006 (68).

Low adherent or gauze dressings

These dressings are characterized by good availability and low material expense. They have a tendency to adhere to the wound resulting in more painful dressing changes and leaving behind microfibers, activating irritation and infection in the wound bed - a disadvantage for this dressing material.

Semi occlusive dressings

Semi occlusive dressings are impermeable to fluids but permit passage of gas molecules. They are suitable to cover freshly closed incisions and enhance epithelialization, but should not be used in contaminated wounds or wounds with moderate or higher exudation.

Hydrogels and hydrocolloids

Hydrogels are complex polysaccharides that maintain a moist wound bed and rehydrate wounds to avoid desiccation. They are non-adhesive and easily detach with dressing changes, as well as being able to absorb moderate amounts of exudate. They can be used in infected wounds, but require a secondary dressing.

Hydrocolloids consist of hydrophilic polymers dispersed in water and are able to absorb mild amounts of exudates while being impermeable to liquids or gases (69). They provide a moist environment but should not be used in heavily colonized or highly exudating wounds.

Foam dressings

Foam dressings are made of non-adhering polyurethane. They are highly absorptive and useful for exudative wounds, but not for non- or minimally exudating wounds. One of the only disadvantages of polyurethane foam dressings is uncontrolled leakage (13, 69).

Alginate dressing

Alginate dressings are naturally occurring amylaceous polysaccharides, extracted from brown seaweed. They are capable of absorbing significant amounts of exudate, but are not qualified for non-exudating wounds. They can absorb 20 times their dry weight and so reduce the necessity of multiple dressings, and if used for dry wounds to maintain wound moisture, they should be hydrated with sterile saline.

Foams, polymers, hydrogles, alginates and hydrocolloids are occlusive wound dressings.

Antimicrobial dressings

This dressing material contains an antimicrobial agent, usually silver. Silver ionized in the moist environment has biologic activity for a broad spectrum of bacteria and against a broad range of microorganisms including highly resistant organisms such as VRE (vancomycin resistant Enterococcus) and MRSA (multi resistant Staphylococcus aureus).

Biosynthetic skin substitute dressings

This dressing material mimics the function of skin by replacing the epidermis and dermis. They allow re-epithelialization and permit gas and fluid exchange.

3. MATERIALS, PATIENTS AND METHODS

3.1 Study Design and Patient Selection

This observational, prospective randomized clinical trial was performed to compare three different dressing materials for donor site wounds in elderly patients receiving split-thickness skin grafts. The study was carried out between July 2012 and June 2013 at the Division of Plastic, Aesthetic and Reconstructive Surgery, Department of Surgery, at the Medical University of Graz. It was approved by the local ethics committee and informed consent was obtained from each patient enrolled in the study. Only patients aged 55 or older were included in the study cohort. Comorbidities like vascular disease, diabetes, and hypertension, as well as carcinoma and smoking habits, were recorded as important variables in this study. Patients were randomly assigned to treatment of the donor site wound with Biatain Ibu (B) Mepilex Ag (M) or Suprathel dressing (S). A detailed description of the dressing material is given below. Patients with high risk for infection, serious disease or systemic medication as well as patients under immunosuppression or radiation therapy were excluded. Size of the expected donor site, gender of the patient and the decision to perform a split-thickness graft were not considered as outcome variables.

Forty-eight patients (26 male, 22 female) were included in the study (n=48). Mean age was 70.9 years (range 55-87). Comorbidities and smoking habits of the patient cohort are presented in Table 1.

Dressing material	Smoking Habits		Comorbidity							
	Nicotine		Diabetes		Tumor		Vascular Disease		Hypertension	
	n	(%)	n	(%)	n	(%)	n	(%)	n	(%)
Biatain Ibu n: 18	5	27.8	5	27.8	6	33.3	5	27.8	11	61.1
Mepilex Ag n:15	4	26.6	5	33.3	6	40	11	73.3	8	53.3
Suprathel n: 15	3	20	2	13.3	3	20	5	33.3	8	53.3
Elderly patient cohort (n:48)	**12**	**25**	**12**	**25**	**15**	**31.3**	**21**	**43.8**	**27**	**56.3**

Table 1. Percentage of smoking habits and comorbidity

3.2 Dressing Materials

Biatain Ibu (B), Mepilex Ag (M) and Suprathel (S) were used as dressing materials in this study. All three dressings are purely synthetic and have special properties that support the moist wound theory. They are easy to handle and adapt to the skinsurface, ensuring an almost painless dressing change guaranteeing minimal interaction until removal of the dressing. The products are available in different sizes.

Patients were randomly assigned to receive one of the aforementioned dressing materials on the donor site wound. A detailed description of the dressing subgroups is given in Table 2.

Biatain Ibu

Biatain Ibu is a nonadhesive foam dressing (Coloplast A/S, Humlebaek, Denmark) consisting of an advanced foam with incorporated ibuprofen. Ibuprofen belongs to a class of drugs called non-steroidal anti-inflammatory drugs (NSAIDs) and is used for the management of mild to moderate pain, fever and inflammation. It is released in the body by prostaglandins, unsaturated carboxylic acids based on the fatty acid arachidonic acid that act as chemical messengers. Ibuprofen inhibits cyclooxygenase, the promotor of prostaglandin, and thus reduces local release of inflammatory mediators. Ibuprofen is distributed in the foam dressing at 0.5mg/cm. Its continuous release is triggered by exudation and regulated by the amount of exsudate from the wound (71).

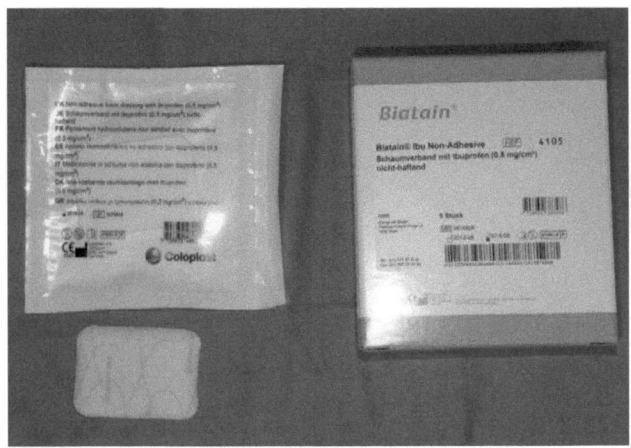

Figure 13. Biatain Ibu (B)

Mepilex Ag

Mepilex Ag (Mölnlicke Healthcare, Sweden) is a soft and highly comfortable anti-microbial foam dressing made from polyurethane foam that absorbs exudate and maintains a moist wound environment. The outer surface of the foam is bound to a vapor-permeable polyurethane membrane, which acts as a barrier to liquid and microorganisms including viruses. The foam contains a silver salt that provides an antimicrobial action, inactivating pathogens taken up by the dressing. The effect is initially detectable within 30 minutes and lasts for up to 7 days. Silver kills bacteria and might be used both for preventing infection and on wounds with signs of local infection. The Safetac-technology ensures that the dressing can be changed without damaging the wound or surrounding skin (72).

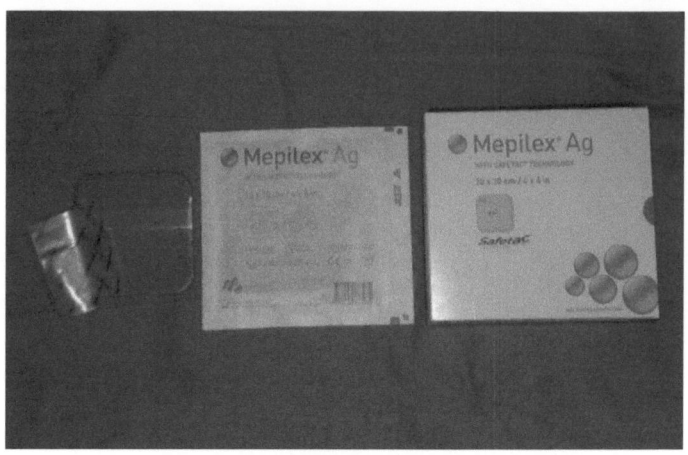

Figure 14. Mepilex Ag (M)

Suprathel

Suprathel (PolyMedics Innovations, Filderstadt, Germany) is an alloplastic copolymer that is able to imitate the properties of natural epithelium by being an absorbable skin substitute that is highly permeable to oxygen and water vapor, and acts as a barrier against germs (bacteria). It mimics an artificial skin substitute with properties of natural epithelium and is considered a temporary skin substitute, primarily engineered/developed for skin graft donor sites in high risk patients, and for burns (73). The membrane adapts instantly to wound surfaces and becomes transparent during the wound healing process, allowing visual control of the healing without any manipulation. The membrane is intended to automatically detach from wound surfaces, which should have a positive impact in terms of pain reduction. Suprathel can be adapted optimally to any body part due to its elastic properties.

Its degradation starts after few days accompanied by a gradual reduction of its permeability to the physiological range of the healthy skin (74).

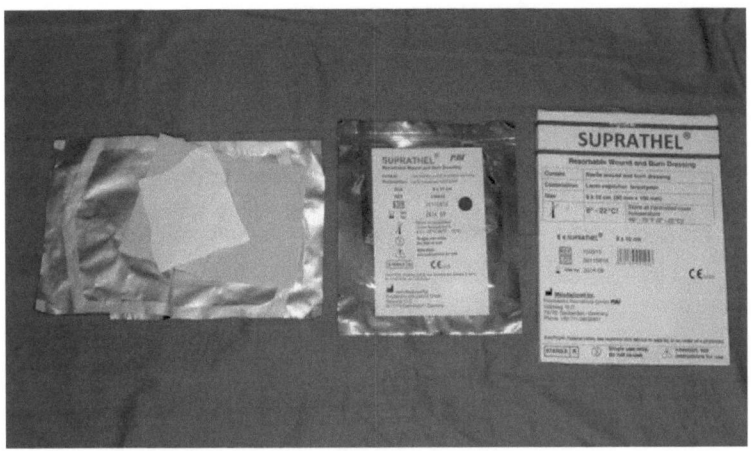

Figure 15. Suprathel (S)

Dressing material	Frequency	Percentage
B	18	37.5
M	15	31.3
S	15	31.3
Total	48	100.0

Table 2. Dressing materials

3.3 Development and Measured Outcome

The split-thickness skin graft was routinely harvested from the anterior lateral or distal part of the thigh with an electrodermatome with an average breadth of 8 mm. The donor sites were postoperatively covered with hydrogen gauzes and patients were randomized to receive Mepilex Ag (M), Suprathel (S) or Biatain Ibu (B) dressing that was applied under sterile conditions at the end of the operation. All patients received standard perioperative pain-treatment. Pain scores were recorded continuously from the first postoperative day and during the first dressing change on the second postoperative day with pain scores before-during-after. Only the superficial gauze layers were removed and renewed at the first dressing change. Two weeks after the operation, the second dressing change was scheduled where all dressing materials were removed and the wound was inspected according to the Hollander Wound Evaluation Scale (HWES). The patients and the medical staff completed the particular standardized questionaires. Photographs of the donor sites were taken. If full re-epithelialization was achieved, no further therapy was necessary otherwise the wound was covered again until complete re-epithelialization was to be expected.

Additional dressing changes were strictly avoided under the study period to minimize manipulation of the donor site wound and decrease pain and discomfort for the patients included. Exceptions were made when bleeding was suspected or patients experienced unexpected pain.

The outcome measurements included:

1. Evaluation of pain level in rest and in movement
2. Re-epithelialization of the donor site
3. Functionality during exercise and acceptability of the dressing (ease of application) – evaluated by the medical/nursing staff and patients
4. Infection and other complications
5. Costs

3.4 Parameter and Tools

3.4.1 Evaluation of pain scores

Pain scores were assessed daily from the first day after operation by using the Visual Analogue Scale (VAS), which is a worldwide recognized scale to quantify pain or discomfort experienced by patients. The patients specify the sensation felt according to a linear scale from 0, indicating no pain, to 10, indicating unbearable pain (75).

We recorded pain scores at rest and in movement and additional pain medication used by patients was noted.

3.4.2 Hollander Wound Evaluation Scale

To determine re-epithelialization of the donor site wound the Hollander Wound Evaluation Scale (HWES, Table.3) was used. The HWES is an objective description of the wound situation to assess erythema, warmth, tenderness and drainage of the wound. No (0) indicating healing, yes (1*; 2*) indicating a prolonged healing duration (1*) or a wound complication such as infection (2*). Donor sites with 75% or more re-epithelialization were categorized as healed.

Hollander Wound Evaluation Scale (objective) after removal of dressing			
Wound description: 10 – 14 d.p. OP			
Erythema	Warmth	Tenderness	Drainage
__No(0)	__No(0)	__No(0)	__No(0)
__Yes(1)	__Yes(1)	__Yes(1)	__Yes(1)
__mm	__mm	__mm	__Purulent(2*)
			__Serosanguineous(1*)

Table 3. Hollander Wound Evaluation Scale (Original Questionnaire)

3.4.3 Subjective questionnaires for the medical staff and the patients

Questionnaire 1 contained eight questions anwered by the medical staff at the removal of the dressing material. Questions asked related to the removal of the dressing, adherence, abnormalities observed when dressing removed, odors and applicability (Table 4). Answers were categorized into four sections (very good, good, moderate, poor). Included are the original questionnaires in German, as the patient cohort received and responded to them in German (Table 4, Table 5).

Beurteilung des ärztlichen bzw. Plegepersonals 10 bis 14 d postoperativ				
+Abnahme des Verbandes	sehr gut	gut	mäßig	schlecht
+Auffälligkeiten nach Abnahme	keine	Wunde blutet	Verband eingetrocknet	Wunde blutet/Verband eingetrocknet
+Entfernen des Produktes von der Wunde	sehr gut	gut	mäßig	schlecht
+Patientenfreundlichkeit	sehr gut	gut	mäßig	schlecht
+Verfärbung/Verschmutzung des Verbandes bzw. der Umgebung (Kleidung,Bett)	keine	gering	mäßig	schlecht
+Geruchsbildung der Wunde	keine	gering	mäßig	stark
+Anwendung/Applizierbarkeit des Testprodukt	sehr einfach	einfach	schwierig	sehr schwierig
+Haftung des Studienmaterials auf der Wunde	sehr gut	gut	mäßig	schlecht

Table 4. Questionnaire 1

Questionnaire 2 evaluated the different dressing materials by the patients. They were asked to answer five questions concerning skin sensation after receiving the dressing material, including questions regarding the nature of the sensation, the tolerance of the skin (e.g. reddening), possible discoloration and overall assessment (Table 5).

Beurteilungsparameter durch Patienten: 10 bis 14 d postoperativ				
+Hautempfinden nach dem Auftragen des Verbandsmaterials	sehr gut	gut	neutral	unangenehm
+Art der Hautempfindung	angenehm	keine	mäßig	schlecht
+Verträglichkeit auf der Haut bzw. Hautrötung	sehr gut	gut	mäßig	schlecht
+Verfärbung/Verschmutizung des Verbandes bzw. der Umgebung (Kleid, Bett)	keine	gering	mäßig	stark
+Gesamtbeurteilung	sehr gut	gut	mäßig	schlecht

Table 5. Questionnaire 2

Grading was sectioned in excellent (0), good (1), neutral/moderate (2) or poor (3).

Low grades were indicative of a good outcome - the higher the grade the worse the outcome and the evaluation.

3.4.4 Photographs

Photographs were taken at the time of dressing-removal to document the re-epithelialization rate of the donor site wound.

3.5   Statistical Methods

The statistical analysis was performed using the Statistical Package for Social Sciences version 15.0 (SPSS Inc., Chicago, IL, USA). Significance was defined as p-value<0.05.
The VAS data are not normally distributet, therefore the median was calculated. The Spearman's rank correlation coefficient (Spearman's rho) is used to measure the statistical dependence between two variables using a monotonic function. It is appropriate for both continuous and discrete variables, including ordinal variables (76).

For re-epithelialization, ease of use and application, as well as patient satisfaction, Fisher's exact test or analysis of variance (ANOVA) was used to evaluate the statistical significance (77).

4. RESULTS

4.1 Pain Levels

Pain scores were recorded continuously from the first postoperative day to the removal of the dressing by the study patients, at rest (VASr) and in movement (VASm), from the first postoperative day to removal.

Biatain Ibu showed statistically significant pain reduction at rest (p<0.001; Table 6) as well as in movement (p<0.026; Table 7).

Correlations

			VAS_day	VAS_at rest
Spearman's rho	VAS_day	Correlation Coefficient	1,000	-,299(**)
		Sig. (2-tailed)	.	,000
		N	252	252
	VAS_at rest	Correlation Coefficient	-,299(**)	1,000
		Sig. (2-tailed)	,000	.
		N	252	252

** Correlation is significant at the 0.01 level (2-tailed).

Table 6. Pain measurement according the VAS for Biatain Ibu at rest (VASr)

Correlations

			VAS_in movement	VAS_day
Spearman's rho	VAS_in movement	Correlation Coefficient	1,000	-,140(*)
		Sig. (2-tailed)	.	,026
		N	252	252
	VAS_day	Correlation Coefficient	-,140(*)	1,000
		Sig. (2-tailed)	,026	.
		N	252	252

* Correlation is significant at the 0.05 level (2-tailed).

Table 7. Pain levels according to VAS for Biatain Ibu in movement (VASm)

A statistically significant pain reduction was also shown for Suprathel at rest (p<0.004; Table 8) and in movement (p<0.002; Table 9).

			VAS_day	VAS_at rest
Spearman's rho	VAS_day	Correlation Coefficient	1,000	-,196(**)
		Sig. (2-tailed)	.	,004
		N	210	210
	VAS_at rest	Correlation Coefficient	-,196(**)	1,000
		Sig. (2-tailed)	,004	.
		N	210	210

** Correlation is significant at the 0.01 level (2-tailed).

Table 8. Pain levels for Suprathel at rest (VASr)

			VAS_in movement	VAS_day
Spearman's rho	VAS_in movement	Correlation Coefficient	1,000	-,215(**)
		Sig. (2-tailed)	.	,002
		N	210	210
	VAS_day	Correlation Coefficient	-,215(**)	1,000
		Sig. (2-tailed)	,002	.
		N	210	210

** Correlation is significant at the 0.01 level (2-tailed)

Table 9. Pain levels for Suprathel in movement (VASm)

However, no significant pain reduction was observed in the patient group with Mepilex Ag (VASr p=0.533; VASm p=0.899) as following tables show.

Correlations

			VAS_day	VAS_at rest
Spearman's rho	VAS_day	Correlation Coefficient	1,000	-,041
		Sig. (2-tailed)	.	,553
		N	210	210
	VAS_at rest	Correlation Coefficient	-,041	1,000
		Sig. (2-tailed)	,553	.
		N	210	210

Table 10. Pain levels for Mepilex Ag at rest (VASr)

Correlations

			VAS_in movemen	VAS_day
Spearman's rho	VAS_in movement	Correlation Coefficient	1,000	,009
		Sig. (2-tailed)	.	,899
		N	210	210
	VAS_day	Correlation Coefficient	,009	1,000
		Sig. (2-tailed)	,899	.
		N	210	210

Table 11. Pain levels for Mepilex Ag in movement (VASm)

Median values of the pain level at rest and in movement are given in Table 12. No difference in the median was observed for pain levels at rest in all three dressing groups. For pain in movement Suprathel showed the highest deviation, whereas Biatain Ibu showed the lowest.

Case Summaries

Dressing material		VAS_at rest	VAS_in movement
B	N	252	252
	Median	,00	,00
M	N	210	210
	Median	,00	,50
S	N	210	210
	Median	,00	1,00
Total	N	672	672
	Median	,00	,00

Table 12. Median values according to pain for the three dressing materials

The detailed statistical analysis of the subgroups is given in the supplement section (Table 20 to Table 25).

4.1.1 Additional pain medication

Six patients (12.5% of the study population) required additional pain medication during the first postoperative days: three patients with Suprathel dressing and three with Mepilex Ag. Two patients with Mepilex dressing did not require the pain medication until the 6th day postoperatively, and then for a 5-day duration; thus they required the greatest amount of medication.

As pain medication, Metamizol (3 g per event, as tablet or drops, mostly 3 times a day, for 3 days at the longest), Paracetamol (0.5 g a day, once a day for 5 days), and Piritramid (7.5 mg, for 3 days, in addition to 2 g Metamizol and Metamizol drops for 5 days) was offered to the patients, according to the pain (Table 13). Paracetamol and Metamizol are non-opioid analgesics and have analgesic, antispasmodic, antipyretic (for Paracetamol) and minimal anti-inflammatory properties (for Metamizol); they are used for the treatment of acute pain mainly after surgery. Piritramid is a synthetic opioid with strong analgesic power (78).

45

		Additonal pain medication		
Patients n (%)	Dressing material	Medication	Amount in g/mg	Duration in average
3 (6.25)	Mepilex Ag	Metamizol Paracetamol (both NSARs) Piritramid (synthetic opioid)	3g/event and drops 0.5g a day 7.5mg/day	5 days for 2 times 2 to 3 days (2 times)
3 (6.25)	Suprathel	Metamizol (NSAR)	3g/event and drops	2 days
0	Biatain Ibu	0	0	0
6 (12.5)				
Total (n:48)				

Table 13. Additional medication required due to the donor site

4.2 Re-epithelialization

The re-epithelialization rate in percent of the donor site wound was assessed when dressing materials were removed. 55.6% of the patients in the Biatain Ibu dressing group showed full re-epithelialization at the time where the dressing was removed (22.2% was half re-epithelialized at this point in time), compared to 67% re-epithelialization of the Mepilex Ag patient cohort (where 13% was 50% re-epithelialized).
Donor site areas treated with Suprathel showed a 60% rate of full re-epithelialization (compared to 20% to 50% each epithelialization of the wound surface).

44.4% of the patients using Biatain Ibu, 40% of the patients with Suprathel and 33% of the Mepilex Ag-dressing-group had re-epithelialization periods longer than 14 days.
A detailed description of the re-epithelialization rates in percentage is provided in Table 14.

Re-epithelialization at time of removal						
	Dressing material					
	Biatain Ibu (n 18)		**Mepilex Ag** (n 15)		**Suprathel** (n 15)	
Re-epithelialized donor site area	n	(%)	n	(%)	n	(%)
Less than 50%	4	22.2	3	20	3	20
50% re-epithelialized	4	22.2	2	13	3	20
75% (=fully re-epithelialized)	**10**	**55.6**	**10**	**67**	**9**	**60**
Total	18	100	15	100	15	100

Table 14. Percentage of re-epithelialization

No statistically significant difference existed in the re-epithelialization rate between all three dressings used in this study (p=0.90; Table 15).

Descriptives

HWE-total

	N	Mean	Std. Deviation	Std. Error	95% Confidence Interval for Mean		Minimum	Maximum
					Lower Bound	Upper Bound		
B	18	1,39	1,195	,282	,79	1,98	0	3
M	15	1,47	1,060	,274	,88	2,05	0	3
S	15	1,27	1,335	,345	,53	2,01	0	3
Total	48	1,38	1,178	,170	1,03	1,72	0	3

ANOVA

HWE-total

	Sum of Squares	df	Mean Square	F	Sig.
Between Groups	,306	2	,153	,106	,900
Within Groups	64,944	45	1,443		
Total	65,250	47			

Table 15. Re-epithelialization (mean ±SD)

Donor site wounds were photographed when the dressing was removed to document re-epithelialization. Figure 16 to Figure 18 illustrate donor sites which are representative for one of the dressing materials used in this study.

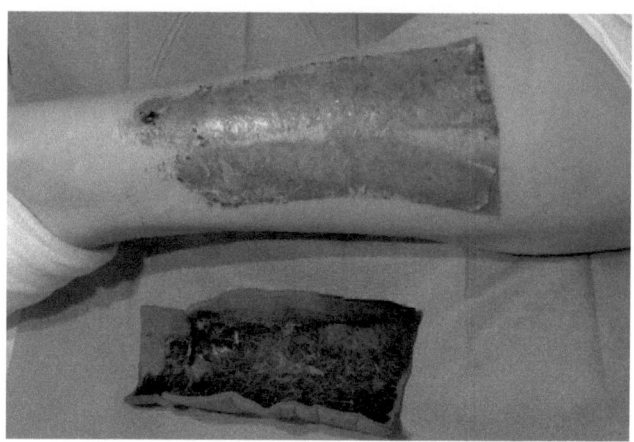

Figure 16. Re-epithelialized donor site 14 days after surgery, dressed with Mepilex Ag

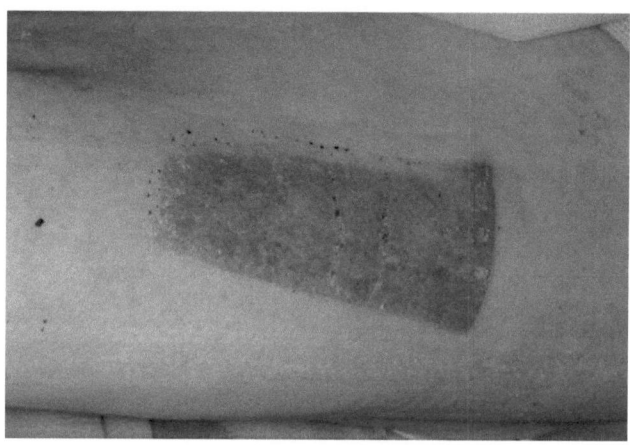

Figure 17. Re-epithelialized donor site 13 days after surgery, dressed with Biatain Ibu

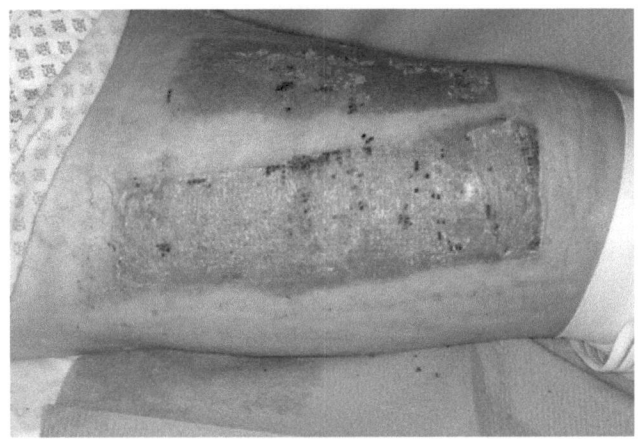

Figure 18. Re-epithelialized donor site 14 days after surgery, dressed with Suprathel

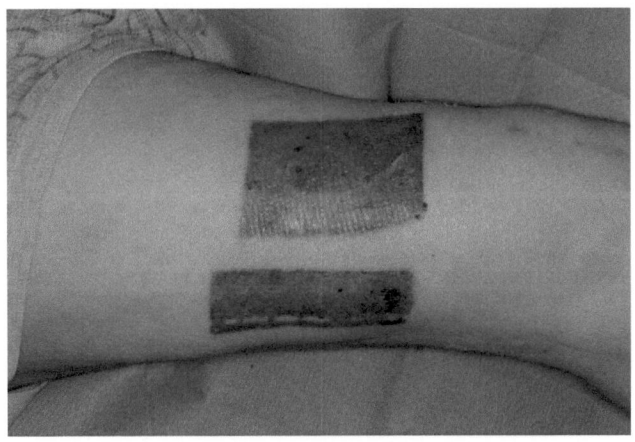

Figure 19. Incompletely re-epithelialized donor site 14 days after surgery, dressed with Suprathel

4.3 Apparent Complications

We observed a hypergranulation and increased pain at one donor site dressed with Mepilex Ag when we removed the foam dressing, where the healing time was prolonged to one month, with frequent dressing changes. The patient did not indicate discomfort or pain until removal of the dressing. Medication was not necessary.

4.4 Ease of Application and Use

All three dressings were easy to handle and apply with good adherence to the wound surface. All of them are available in different sizes and by covering only the wound bed they prevent maceration entirely.

Questionnaires filled in by the medical staff were evaluated and detailed data are shown in Table 16. Mepilex Ag dressing was removed easily in over 90% of the patients (classified as excellent and good) followed by Suprathel (68%) and Biatain Ibu (44%). However, 80% of all patients in the Mepilex group experienced problems after dressing removal (classified as moderate and poor). Mepilex Ag was most easy to remove from the wound surface followed by Suprathel and Biatain Ibu. No significant differences were recorded regarding pleasantness for the patient, off odors and application of the dressing material. Discoloration of the dressings did occur more frequently in the Mepilex Ag group compared with the other dressings used in this study.

		Dressing material					
		Biatain Ibu n (18)		Mepilex Ag n (15)		Suprathel n (15)	
		n	(%)	n	(%)	n	%
Dressing removal	Excellent	3	16.7	5	33.3	3	20.0
	Good	5	27.7	9	60.0	7	46.7
	Moderate	7	38,9	1	6.7	1	6.6
	Poor	3	16.7	0	0	4	26.7
	Total	18	100	15	100	15	100
Noticeable problems after dressing removal	Excellent	5	27.7	2	13.3	6	40.0
	Good	3	16.7	1	6.7	0	0
	Moderate	7	38.9	5	33.3	4	26.7
	Poor	3	16.7	7	46.7	5	33.3
	Total	18	100	15	100	15	100
Removal from the wound surface	Excellent	2	11.1	4	26.7	1	6.6
	Good	5	27.8	10	66.7	7	46.7
	Moderate	9	50	1	6.6	4	26.7
	Poor	2	11.1	0	0	3	20
	Total	18	100	15	100	15	100
Pleasantness for the patient	Excellent	10	55.6	13	86.	8	53.3
	Good	8	44.4	2	13.3	6	40
	Moderate	0	0	0	0	1	6.7
	Poor	0	0	0	0	0	0
	Total	18	100	15	100	15	100
Mess or discoloration in proximity	Excellent	14	77.8	12	80	14	93.3
	Good	4	22.2	1	6.7	1	6.7
	Moderate	0	0	2	13.3	0	0
	Poor	0	0	0	0	0	0
	Total	18	100	15	100	15	100
Off odors	Excellent	14	77.8	10	66.7	13	86.6
	Good	2	11.1	4	26.6	1	6.7
	Moderate	2	11.1	1	6.7	1	6.7
	Poor	0	0	0	0	0	0
	Total	18	100	15	100	15	100
Application of the dressing material	Excellent	13	72.2	11	73.3	11	73.3
	Good	5	27.8	4	26.6	4	26.7
	Moderate	0	0	0	0	0	0
	Poor	0	0	0	0	0	0
	Total	18	100	15	100	15	100
Adherence to the wound bed	Excellent	8	44.4	6	40	8	53.3
	Good	9	50	9	60	7	46.7
	Moderate	1	5.6	0	0	0	0
	Poor	0	0	0	0	0	0
	Total	18	100	15	100	15	100

Table 16. Evaluation by the medical staff

No statistically significant difference for ease of use and application was apparent as between all three dressings used in this study (p=0.69; Table17).

Descriptives

BeurÄ.ges

	N	Mean	Std. Deviation	Std. Error	95% Confidence Interval for Mean		Minimum	Maximum
					Lower Bound	Upper Bound		
B	18	6,28	2,866	,675	4,85	7,70	1	13
M	15	5,40	2,558	,660	3,98	6,82	0	9
S	15	6,07	3,615	,933	4,06	8,07	1	12
Total	48	5,94	2,992	,432	5,07	6,81	0	13

ANOVA

Ease of use and application

	Sum of Squares	Df	Mean Square	F	Sig.
Between Groups	6,668	2	3,334	,362	,698
Within Groups	414,144	45	9,203		
Total	420,813	47			

Table 17. Statistical analysis for ease of use and application (mean ±SD)

4.5 Patient Satisfaction

Evaluation of questionaire 2, which was completed by patients, showed a high level of satisfaction with all dressing types used in this study. Skin sensation after application of the dressing (classified as moderate and poor) was most frequent in the Suprathel group (more than 50%) followed by Biatain Ibu (44%) and Mepilex Ag (40%). Only 7% of patients in the Suprathel group experienced discoloration compared to 17% in the Biatain Ibu group and 13% in the Mepilex AG group. Interestingly, 20% of patients in the Suprathel group evaluated the applied dressing as moderate and poor in the overall assessment, followed by 7% in the Mepilex dressing category. All patients in the Biatain dressing evaluated the dressing as excellent and good (Table 18).

		Dressing material					
		Biatain Ibu n (18)		Mepilex Ag n (15)		Suprathel n (15)	
		n	(%)	n	(%)	n	(%)
Skin sensation after receiving the dressing material	Excellent	2	11.2	3	20.0	1	6.8
	Good	8	44.4	6	40	6	40
	Moderate	8	44.4	5	33.3	4	26.6
	Poor	0	0	1	6.7	4	26.6
	Total	18	100	15	100	15	100
Type of skin sensation	Excellent	3	16.7	0	0	2	13.3
	Good	11	61.1	6	40	6	40
	Moderate	4	22.2	9	60	4	26.7
	Poor	0	0	0	0	3	20
	Total	18	100	15	100	15	100
Tolerance for the skin e.g. reddening	Excellent	10	58.8	9	60	6	40
	Good	8	41.2	6	40	7	46.7
	Moderate	0	0	0	0	2	13.3
	Poor	0	0	0	0	0	0
	Total	18	100	15	100	15	100
Possible discoloration (clothes, bed)	Excellent	14	77.8	10	66.7	11	73.3
	Good	1	5.5	3	20	3	20
	Moderate	1	5.5	2	13.3	1	6.7
	Poor	2	11.2	0	0	0	0
	Total	18	100	15	100	15	100
Overall assessment	Excellent	4	22.2	8	53.3	2	13.3
	Good	14	77.8	6	40	10	66.7
	Moderate	0	0	1	6.7	2	13.3
	Poor	0	0	0	0	1	6.7
	Total	18	100	15	100	15	100

Table 18. Patient evaluation of the dressing materials

No statistically significant difference was shown between all dressing materials as evaluated by the patients (p=0.11; Table 19).

Descriptives

BeurP.ges

	N	Mean	Std. Deviation	Std. Error	95% Confidence Interval for Mean Lower Bound	Upper Bound	Minimum	Maximum
B	18	3,94	1,474	,347	3,21	4,68	0	6
M	15	4,27	2,344	,605	2,97	5,56	1	8
S	15	5,60	3,043	,786	3,92	7,28	1	12
Total	48	4,56	2,387	,345	3,87	5,26	0	12

ANOVA

Patient Evaluation

	Sum of Squares	df	Mean Square	F	Sig.
Between Groups	24,335	2	12,167	2,249	,117
Within Groups	243,478	45	5,411		
Total	267,812	47			

Table 19. ANOVA for patient evalution of dressing material (mean ±SD)

4.6 Cost

The cost for Biatain Ibu is significantly lower than it is for the same size of Mepilex Ag, but both of the artificial foam dressings cost significantly less than the temporary artificial skin replacement Suprathel. Mepilex costs almost twice as much as Biatain, and Suprathel costs almost seven times as much as Biatain does (79). All three highly qualificated wound dressings can stay on place until re-epithelialization.

5. DISCUSSION

Donor site wounds from harvested split-thickness skin grafts (STSG) impose significant pain, irritation and discomfort for patients, so that they are often perceived more disturbing by the patients than the site treated with the graft (14, 80). In a split thickness skin graft study performed on patients with diabetic foot ulcers 60% in the control group turned down the option of skin grafting because they did not want to have another painful wound (81) showing that pain plays a key role in fragile patient groups burdened with comorbidities like diabetes or cardiovascular diseases.

Although numerous studies have been performed to find the optimal dressing for donor site wounds there is still no consensus (14, 79, 82). The optimal dressing material should reduce pain and avoid leakage of exudate, enhance epithelialization and provide the greatest patient comfort, as well as be easily handled and economical in cost (3, 81). Modern dressing materials like semi-occlusive and occlusive dressings fulfill these criteria by creating a moist wound healing environment, especially for high risk wound care (81, 82).

All three dressing materials used in this study meet the requirements of modern wound management. They support the natural healing process and show good acceptability by patients. We observed a statistically significant pain reduction in the Biatain Ibu and Surathel group which is in line with findings by other autors (3, 79). They observed an immediate pain relief after application of Biatain due to the incorporated ibuprofen (3). In our study patients with Suprathel dressing experienced slight pain at the beginning of the study period, however, the pain decreased gradually over time, which is in contrast to Markls observation of renewed pain after five days in the patient group with Suprathel (3). Interestingly, all patients assigned to the Mepilex Ag group showed high satisfaction with the dressing material at the beginning of the study, but complained of pain or discomfort, mainly in movement in the second half of the study-period. This observation is in accordance with data published by Kaartinen et al which show a significant difference in pain levels between patients with Suprathel dressing compared to the patients in the Mepilex group (79). We hypothesize that this observation in our study may have been induced by a scab that became bound to the foam, which induced irritation and reactivated bleeding when the foam was loosened and thus resulted in pain and discomfort as healing progressed. We could not observe a statistically significant pain reduction in the Mepilex Ag group and one can only speculate whether the incorporated silver ions decreased pain in this patient group in the first half of the study period (83).

Only six patients included in this study requested additional pain medication, however, all these patients already had severe wounds before and it might have been difficult for them to localize the exact source of their pain.

In terms of re-epithelialization, there was no noteworthy difference between the dressing materials compared, in line with other studies (3, 70). In fact, it may not be possible, even with the best dressing materials, to greatly shorten the healing process. Early removal of the dressing should be strictly avoided as it will disturb the re-epithelialization process that already has occurred. Although dressing changes and removals in this study were carried out with minimal intervention the adhesion property of the dressing materials was an important key factor. Biatain Ibu dressing adhered best to the wound surface but was the one most difficult to detach from the wound area followed by Mepilex Ag. Both dressing materials are polyurethane films that lose their adherence when the wound healing process is completed. However, if a scab adhered to the dressing – most often in the centre of the dressing, but also at the peripheral wound margins – the patients complained of greater discomfort and pain. This was observed at the end of the study-period most noticeably with Mepilex Ag. Otherwise the polyurethane dressings fulfilled their properties to provide an ideal healing environment and felt confortable to the patients, reducing or preventing pain, limiting shearing forces and minimizing labor input significantly (14, 70) by being kept in place until complete epithelialization.

It was more challenging to remove dressings from large wound areas, and the healing result of a continuous dressing piece was better than when the wound bed was covered with two separate dressing-parts, which resulted in irregular wound healing. By soaking the dressing with 3% hydrogen peroxide, or with 0.9% sodium chloride, loosening of the dressing was improved. Suprathel was the dressing with the best bonding, because it is thinner and conforms to the body shape. It also directs exudate into the outer gauze dressing rather than absorbing it. Suprathel dissolves during the healing process, but when the gauze and the scab merged, Suprathel thus adhered most to the wound which made it the most difficult to replace. As Suprathel becomes transparent while the healing process continues, it should allow the wound surface to be visible. Although it is designed for this purpose, we could not confirm whether sight of the wound surface was possible because the Suprathel had stuck to the paraffin gauze and by separating the superficial gauze, we provoked renewed bleeding. This insufficient material transparency of Suprathel was also discussed by Markl et al (3). Its semitransparent characteristic might be of importance when there are larger wound beds, such as in burn patients in respect of whom Suprathel is well researched (79, 80). By observing these problems we removed the dressing in some patients the earliest on day 14 postoperatively, where full re-epithelialization was expected to minimize bleeding risk and painful dressing removal. Interestingly, Kaartinen and Kuokkanen reported that Suprathel inhibited bleedings in donor sites and they did not discuss any problems with the onlying dressing layers to Suprathel (79). We observed in our study enhanced postoperative bleedings with Suprathel, which required additional gauze layers and occasionally more superficial dressing changes.

In comparison to Suprathel, the foam dressings loosened from the epithelialized wound area and became stiff over the course of the time (Fig. 15). Foam dressings possess absorptive capacity, which is not unlimited and depends on the wound dimension (14), whereas Suprathel acts by loading exudate into the outer dressings. With large donor sites we observed that the intake capacity was at its limit, but it was not a handicap to the healing process. Heavy postoperative bleeding detaches the dressing from the wound surface and reduces the effect of the dressing (17). We did not observe uncontrolled leakage in the foam dressing groups, an often-described disadvantage of this dressing (76, 77).

However, a limitation in this study is the difficulty in estimating the exact re-epithelialization time, as all dressings were removed when the epithelialization process was expected to be complete. Läuchli et al performed a randomized controlled trial comparing a calcium alginate dressing versus a polyurethane dressing the authors also discussed this shortcoming of their study (80).

Patients in all three study subgroups were highly content with the dressing types received. Uncomfortable skin sensations were recorded more frequently in the Suprathel group, however, the fear of exudate leakage and soiling of clothes and bed linen was lowest in this group and highest in the foam dressing groups; this is in line with findings by other authors (80). All three dressings had easy application and handling, as well as similar levels of patient comfort and satisfaction. Some of the patients had past experience in split-thickness skin therapy and subjectively were highly satisfied with these new comfortable dressing products.

Although the study population comprised elderly patients with high risk comorbidities prone to infection, there was no wound infection recorded. Mepilex Ag, as a silver-containing dressing for donor sites as well as for burns, has broad-spectrum antimicrobial properties with rapid and sustained action – according to Silverstein et al less analgesia is necessary with Mepilex Ag, which should prevent complications like infection, while automatically featuring pain reduction (83). Silver dressings show good results in clinical studies (2, 81) but do not surpass other highly qualified dressings (81, 83, 84). It is unresolved whether the advantages result only from the effect of the silver ions, or from the high performance of the foam dressing. The Mepilex Ag patient group was painless in the first half of the study time, but complained problems in the second. It is possible that this problem could be solved with an additional dressing change, which would, however, interrupt the healing process and require greater effort with higher costs. Due to the limited size of our patient cohort, we can only make observations rather than draw conclusions, and thus cannot contradict the findings of similar studies.

Even though the costs for the dressing material used in this study in average are high (3, 79, 81), it is still economical as the dressings provide the best support in wound healing, are easy in handling and provide a high comfort for the patients (85). All three dressing are available in different sizes, are conformable to the body's surface and are labour and cost efficient due to the minimal interaction required until removal of the dressing (85). Markl reported complex and time-consuming dressing changes with Mepithel and Biatain Ibu. In addition, patients today need not remain hospitalized until dressing removal.

6. CONCLUSIONS

Maintenance for donor site wounds in STSG patients is a complex task and comprises not only the perioperative wound management but the whole healing phase. The "ideal wound dressing" always depends upon the patient's individual demands, and in that respect, polyurethane dressings - especially Biatain Ibu - would fulfill the criteria of an ideal donor site dressing. Although an ideal dressing does not yet exist, the polymer foams and Suprathel guarantee a supportive and painless healing-process with low intervention, especially in high-risk patients, and thus meet the requirements of an ideal dressing. It is impossible to meet all of the requirements of an ideal dressing isochronally, because there are different focuses at particular points in time. We observed painlessness as most important for patients immediately after surgery, as well as a painless dressing removal prior to re-epithelialization.

Suprathel was engineered as a dressing to cover donor sites after split-thickness skin transplantation (73). There should be no compromise in giving the patient the best possible individual care, but it is also a responsibility of medical care taker to consider the economic aspects. With respect to the higher cost and compared to the two foam dressings, it is not necessary to choose the most expensive one for the donor site, even in high-risk patients: more expensive does not always mean the best.

We can further conclude that even though the costs for the dressing material used in this study are high on average, it is still economical as they provide the best support in wound healing, are easy to handle and provide high patient comfort. Subjectively, patients who had foam dressings appeared more satisfied.
From an observational perspective, there was no significant difference in the characteristics of the three dressing materials (particularly the foam dressings) but we found that the discomfort caused to the patient at the donor site was negligible in comparison with the preoperative wound situation which is the primary aim and purpose in STSG donor site wound management.

7. SUPPLEMENT

7.1 Statistical Analysis (Complete Data)

Pain levels:

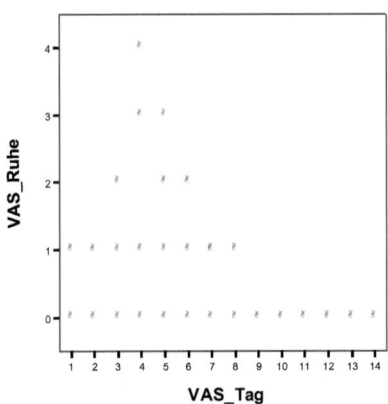

Correlations

			VAS_day	VAS_at rest
Spearman's rho	VAS_day	Correlation Coefficient	1,000	-,299(**)
		Sig. (2-tailed)	.	,000
		N	252	252
	VAS_at rest	Correlation Coefficient	-,299(**)	1,000
		Sig. (2-tailed)	,000	.
		N	252	252

** Correlation is significant at the 0.01 level (2-tailed).

Table 20. Pain measurement according the VAS for Biatain Ibu at rest

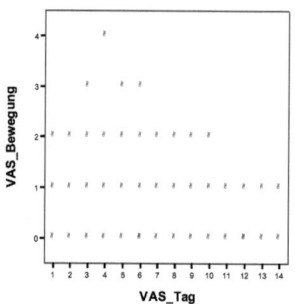

Correlations

			VAS_in movement	VAS_day
Spearman's rho	VAS_in movement	Correlation Coefficient	1,000	-,140(*)
		Sig. (2-tailed)	.	,026
		N	252	252
	VAS_day	Correlation Coefficient	-,140(*)	1,000
		Sig. (2-tailed)	,026	.
		N	252	252

* Correlation is significant at the 0.05 level (2-tailed).

Table 21. Pain levels according to VAS for Biatain Ibu in movement

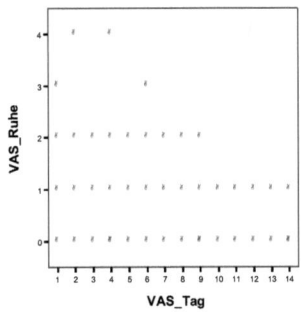

Correlations

			VAS_day	VAS_at rest
Spearman's rho	VAS_day	Correlation Coefficient	1,000	-,196(**)
		Sig. (2-tailed)	.	,004
		N	210	210
	VAS_at rest	Correlation Coefficient	-,196(**)	1,000
		Sig. (2-tailed)	,004	.
		N	210	210

** Correlation is significant at the 0.01 level (2-tailed).

Table 22. Pain levels for Suprathel at rest

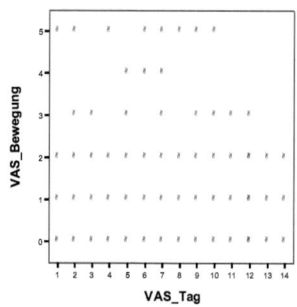

Correlations

			VAS_in movement	VAS_day
Spearman's rho	VAS_in movement	Correlation Coefficient	1,000	-,215(**)
		Sig. (2-tailed)	.	,002
		N	210	210
	VAS_day	Correlation Coefficient	-,215(**)	1,000
		Sig. (2-tailed)	,002	.
		N	210	210

** Correlation is significant at the 0.01 level (2-tailed)

Table 23. Pain levels for Suprathel in movement

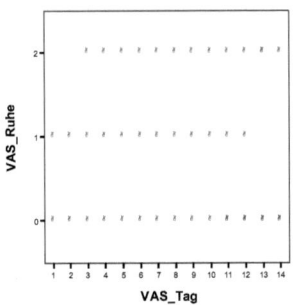

Correlations

			VAS_day	VAS_at rest
Spearman's rho	VAS_day	Correlation Coefficient	1,000	-,041
		Sig. (2-tailed)	.	,553
		N	210	210
	VAS_at rest	Correlation Coefficient	-,041	1,000
		Sig. (2-tailed)	,553	.
		N	210	210

Table 24. Pain levels for Mepilex Ag at rest; with no statistical significance

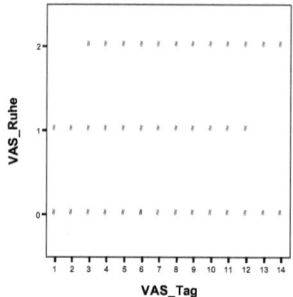

Correlations

			VAS_in movement	VAS_day
Spearman's rho	VAS_in movement	Correlation Coefficient	1,000	,009
		Sig. (2-tailed)	.	,899
		N	210	210
	VAS_day	Correlation Coefficient	,009	1,000
		Sig. (2-tailed)	,899	.
		N	210	210

Table 25. Pain levels for Mepilex Ag in movement; with no statistical significance

8. REFERENCES

1. Kelton PL. Skin grafting. Sel Readings Plast Surg. 1999;9(1):1–10.

2. Bailey S, Carmean M, Cinat M, Burton K, Lane C, Malinoski D. A Randomized Comparison Study of Aquacel Ag and Glucan II as Donor Site Dressings With Regard to Healing Time, Cosmesis, Infection Rate, and Patient's Perceived Pain: A Pilot Study. J Burn Care Res. 2011;(32):627–32.

3. Markl P, Prantl L, Schreml S, Babilas P, Landthaler M, Schwarze H. Management of split-thickness donor sites with synthetic wound dressings: results of a comparative clinical study. Ann Plast Surg. 2010;65:490–6.

4. Wood RJ, Peltier GL, Twomey JA. Management of the difficult split-thickness donor site. Ann Plast Surg. 1989;22:80–1.

5. Timmons J. Skin function and wound healing physiology. Wound Essentials. 2006;1.

6. Sieglbauer F. Normale Anatomie des Menschen. 3. Auflage. Urban & Schwarzenberg, Hrsg. Berlin-Wien; 1935.

7. Thornton JF, Gosman AA. Skin Grafts And Skin Substitutes And Principles Of Flaps. Sel Readings Plast Surg. 2004;10(1).

8. Fanhänel J, Pera F, Anderhuber F, Nitsch R, Hrsg. Waldeyer: Anatomie des Menschen. 17. Auflage. Walter de Gruyter Verlag Berlin, New York; 2003.

9. Benninghoff. Anatomie, Makroskopische Anatomie, Embryologie und Histologie des Menschen, Band 2. 16. Auflage. Drenckhahn D, Hrsg. München: Elsevier GmbH, Urban und Fischer; 2004.

10. Ovalle WK, Nahirney PC, editors. Netter's Essential Histology. 2nd Edition. Philadelphia: Elsevier; 2013.

11. Jensen PK, Bolund L. Tissue culture of human epidermal keratinocytes: a differentiating model system for gene testing and somatic gene therapy. J Cell Sci [Internet]. 1991 Oct;100 (Pt 2:255–9. Available from: http://www.ncbi.nlm.nih.gov/pubmed/1757485

12. James WD, Berger TG, Elston DM, editors. Andrew's Diseases of the Skin, Clinical Dermatology. 11th Edition. Elsevier Health Sciences; 2011.

13. No Title [Internet]. Available from: http://kreativestudios.com/Tooltip/05Integument/03dermis.html

14. Dornseifer U, Lonic D, Gerstung TI, Herter F, Fichter AM, Holm C, et al. The ideal split-thickness skin graft donor-site dressing: a clinical comparative trial of a modified polyurethane dressing and aquacel. Plast Reconstr Surg. 2011;128:918–24.

15. Thorne CH, Chung KC, Gosain AK, Gurtner GC, Mehrara GJ, Rubin JP, et al., editors. Grabb & Smith's Plastic Surgery. 7th Edition. Philadelphia: Lippincott, Williams & Wilkins; 2013.

16. Chick LR. Brief history and biology of skin grafting. Ann Plast Surg. 1988;21(4):358–65.

17. Ratner D. Skin grafting: From here to there. Dermatologic Clinics. 1998. p. 75–90.

18. Hauben DJ, Baruchin A, Mahler D. On the History of the Free Skin Graft. Annals of Plastic Surgery. 1982. p. 242–6.

19. Santoni-Rugiu P, Sykes PJ. A History of Plastic Surgery. Schröder G, editor. Springer-Verlag, Berlin Heildelberg; 2007.

20. Reverdin J. Graffe Epidermique. Experience faite dans le service de M. le docteur Guyon a'l hopital Necker. Bull Imp Soc Chir Paris. 1869;10:511–5.

21. Thiersch C. Ueber die feinen anatomischen Veränderungen bei Aufheilung von Haut auf Granulationen. Verhandlungen der Dtsch Gesellschaft für Chir. 1874;(3):69–75.

22. Gabarro P. A New Method of Grafting. Br Med J. 1943;1:723–4.

23. Brown JB, McDowell F. MASSIVE REPAIRS OF BURNS WITH THICK SPLIT-SKIN GRAFTS*. Ann Surg. 1942;115:658–74.

24. Tanner JJ, Vandeput J, Olley J. The mesh skin graft. Plast Reconstr Surg. 1964;34:287–92.

25. Rheinwald, James G, Green H. Serial Cultivation of Strains of Human Epidermal Keratinocytes: the Formation of Keratinizing Colonies from Single Cells. Department of Biology Massachusetts Institute of Technology; 1975. p. 331–44.

26. Rudolph R, Klein L. Healing processes in skin grafts. Surg Gynecol Obs. 1973;

27. Davis J. Adress of the president: the story of plastic surgery. Ann Surg. 1941;113(5):641–113.

28. MacNeil S. Progress and opportunities for tissue-engineered skin. Nature. 2007;455:874–80.

29. Biswas A, Bharara M, Hurst C, Armstrong DG, Rilo H. The micrograft concept for wound healing: strategies and applications. J Diabetes Sci Technol [Internet]. 2010 Jul;4(4):808–19. Available from: http://www.pubmedcentral.nih.gov/articlerender.fcgi?artid=2909510&tool=pmcentre z&rendertype=abstract

30. Beldon P. WHAT YOU NEED TO KNOW ABOUT SKIN GRAFTS AND DONOR SITE WOUNDS. Wound Essentials. 2007;2:149–55.

31. Yang C, Shih T, Chu T, Hsu W, Kuo S, Chao Y. The intermingled transplantation of auto- and homografts in severe burns. Burns. 1980;6(3):151–5.

32. Meek C. Successful microdermagrafting using the Meek-Wall microdermatome. Am JSurg. 1958;96(4):557–8.

33. Meek C. Microdermagrafting - the Meek technic. Hosp Top. 1965;43:114–6.

34. Zhang M, Chang Z, Han X, Zhu M. Microskin grafting. I. Animal experiments. Burn Incl Term Inj. 1986;12(8):540–3.

35. Shevchenko R V, James SL, James SE. R EVIEW A review of tissue-engineered skin bioconstructs available for skin reconstruction. 2010;(October 2009):229–58.

36. Shoemaker PJ. Split Thickness Skin Grafting. Can Fam Physician. 1982;28:1145–7.

37. Rudolph R, Milson T. Species differences in the trypsin separation of epidermis and dermis. Plast Reconstr Surg. 1976;58:459–65.

38. Branham G, Thomas J. Skin grafts: facial plastic surgery. Otolaryngol Clin North Am. 1990;23(5):889–7.

39. Böcker W, Denk H, Heitz PU, Moch H, Höfler G, Kreipe H. Pathologie. 5. Auflage. München: Urban & Fischer; 2012.

40. Converse JM, Smahel J, Ballantyne DL, Harper AD. Inosculation of vessels of skin graft and host bed: a fortuitous encounter. Br J Plast Surg [Internet]. 1975 Oct [cited 2014 Apr 27];28(4):274–82. Available from: http://www.ncbi.nlm.nih.gov/pubmed/1104028

41. Forrest RD. Early history of wound treatment. J R Soc Med. 1982;57.

42. Majno G. The Healing Hand: Man and Wound in the Ancient World. Cambridge: Harvard niversity Press; 1975.

43. Scholl R. Der Papyrus Ebers. Die grösste Buchrolle zur Heilkunde Ägyptens (Schriften aus der Universitäts-Bibliothek Leipzig, Bd 7). Band 7. Leipzig: Universitäts-Bibliothek Leipzig; 2002.

44. Converse JM, Littler JW. Reconstructive Plastic Surgery: Principles and Procedures in Correction, Reconstruction and Transplantation. 3rd Edition. Converse JM, editor. Saunders; 1977.

45. Clark FC. A Brief History of Antiseptic Surgery. Med Library Hist J. 1907;5(3):145–72.

46. Bull J, Squire J, Topley E. Experiments with occlusive dressings of a new plastic. Lancet. 1948;2:213–4.

47. Winter GD. Formation of the scab and the rate of epithelisation of superficial wounds in the skin of the young domestic pig. 1962. J Wound Care. 1995;4:366–367; discussion 368–371.

48. Hinman CD, Maibach H. Effect of air exposure and occlusion on experimental human skin wounds. Nature. 1963;(200):377–8.

49.   Bishop SM, Walker M, Rogers AA, Chen WYJ. Importance of moisture balance at the wound-dressing interface. J Wound Care. 2003;12:125–8.

50.   Cutting KF, White RJ, Butcher M. Wound dressing performance: meeting 21st century requirements. J Wound Care. 2010;20.

51.   Zhao M, Song B, Pu J, Wada T, Reid B, Tai G, et al. Electrical signals control wound healing through phosphatidylinositol-3-OH kinase-gamma and PTEN. Nature. 2006;442:457–60.

52.   Rapid T, Service R, Cadth W. Dressing and Care of Skin Graft Sites. Can Agency Drugs Technol Heal. 2013.

53.   Schultz GS, Sibbald RG, Falanga V, Ayello EA, Dowsett C, Harding K, et al. Wound bed preparation: A systematic approach to wound management. Wound Repair Regen. 2002;11:1–28.

54.   Kelton PJ. Skin grafts and skin substitutes. Sel Readings Plast Surg. 1999;10(1).

55.   Ferguson MWJ, O'Kane S. Scar-free healing: from embryonic mechanisms to adult therapeutic intervention. Philos Trans R Soc Lond B Biol Sci [Internet]. 2004 May 29 [cited 2014 Mar 20];359(1445):839–50. Available from: http://www.pubmedcentral.nih.gov/articlerender.fcgi?artid=1693363&tool=pmcentrez&rendertype=abstract

56.   Whitby DJ, Ferguson MW. The extracellular matrix of lip wounds in fetal, neonatal and adult mice. Development. 1991;112:651–68.

57.   Ferguson M, Whitby D, Shah M, Armstrond D, Siebert W, Longaker M. Scar formation: the spectral nature of fetal and adult wound repair. Plast Reconstr Surg. 1996;97(4):854–60.

58.   Weber RS, Hankins P, Limitone E, Callender D, Frankenthaler RM, Wolf P, et al. Split-thickness skin graft donor site management. A randomized prospective trial comparing a hydrophilic polyurethane absorbent foam dressing with a petrolatum gauze dressing. Archives of otolaryngology--head & neck surgery. 1995 p. 1145–9.

59.   Menaker GM. Wound Dressings for Office-Based Surgery. Facial Plastic Surgery. 2004. p. 91–105.

60.   Giljes O. On taping (adhesive tape treatment) of leg ulcers. Acta Derm Venereol. 1948;28:454–67.

61.   Morgan D. Setting up wound dressing guidelines: avoiding the pitfalls. J Tissue Viability. 1998;8(3):5–8.

62.   Thomas S. Hydrocolloid dressings in the management of acute wounds: a review of the literature. Int Wound J. 2008;5:602–13.

63.   Kloeters O, Schierle C, Tandara A, Mustoe TA. The use of a semi-occlusive dressing reduces epidermal inflammatory cytokine expression and mitigates dermal proliferation and inflammation in a rat incisional model. Wound Repair Regen. 2008;16(4):568–75.

64. Muangman P, Nitimonton S, Aramwit P. Comparative Clinical Study of Bactigras and Telfa AMD for Skin Graft Donor-Site Dressing. International Journal of Molecular Sciences. 2011. p. 5031–8.

65. Allen H, Edgerton M, Rodeheaver C. Skin dressings in the treatment of contaminated wounds. Am J Surg. 1973;126(45).

66. Szabo S, Tomey E, Linn P. Does skin have antimicrobial properties? An in-vitro experiment and literature review. Am Surg. 1978;44(55).

67. Paddle-Ledinek JE, Nasa Z, Cleland HJ. Effect of different wound dressings on cell viability and proliferation. Plast Reconstr Surg. 2006;117:110S–118S; discussion 119S–120S.

68. Jones V, Grey JE, Harding KG. Wound dressings. BMJ. 2006;332:777–80.

69. No Title [Internet]. Available from: http://www.dressings.org/Dressings/granufl-brd.html

70. Dornseifer U, Fichter AM, Herter F, Sturtz G, Ninkovic M. The ideal split-thickness skin graft donor site dressing: rediscovery of polyurethane film. Ann Plast Surg. 2009;63:198–200.

71. No Title [Internet]. Available from: www.coloplast.com

72. No Title [Internet]. Available from: www.molnlycke.com

73. Schwarze H, Küntscher M, Uhlig C, Hierlemann H, Prantl L, Noack N, et al. Suprathel, a new skin substitute, in the management of donor sites of split-thickness skin grafts: Results of a clinical study. Burns. 2007;33:850–4.

74. No Title [Internet]. Available from: www.polymedics.de

75. Reips U-D, Funke F. Interval level measurement with visual analogue sales in Internet-based research: VAS-Generator. 2008.

76. Lehman A. Jmp For Basic Univariate And Multivariate Statistics: A Step-by-step Guide. 2005.

77. Freedman DA. Statistical Models: Theory and Practice, Cambridge University Press. ISBN 978-0-521-67105-7. Cambridge University Press; 2005.

78. Mutschler E, Geisslinger G, Kroemer HK, Schäfer-Kortnig M. Mutschler Arzneimittlwirkungen. Lehrbuch der Pharmakologie und Toxikologie. 8. Auflage. Stuttgart: Wiss. Verl.-Ges.; 2001.

79. Kaartinen IS, Kuokkanen HO. Suprathel causes less bleeding and scarring than Mepilex Transfer in the treatment of donor sites of split-thickness skin grafts. J Plast Surg Hand Surg. 2011;45:200.203.

80. Läuchli S, Hafner J, Ostheeren S, Mayer D, Barysch MJ, French LE. Management of split-thickness skin graft donor sites: A randomized controlled trial of calcium alginate versus polyurethane film dressing. Dermatology. 2014;227:361–6.

81. Mahmoud SM, Mohamed AA, Mahdi SEI, Ahmed ME. Split-skin graft in the management of diabetic foot ulcers. J Wound Care. 2008;17:303–6.

82. Demirtas Y, Yagmur C, Soylemez F, Ozturk N, Demir A. Management of split-thickness skin graft donor site: A prospective clinical trial for comparison of five different dressing materials. Burns. 2010;36:999–1005.

83. Silverstein P, Heimbach D, Meites H, Latenser B, Mozingo D, Mullins F, et al. An Open, Parallel, Randomized, Comparative, Multicenter Study to Evaluate the Cost-Effectiveness, Performance, Tolerance, and Safety of a Silver-Containing Soft Silicone Foam Dressing (Intervention) vs Silver Sulfadiazine Cream. Journal of Burn Care & Research. 2011. p. 617–26.

84. Duteille F, Jeffery SLA. A phase II prospective, non-comparative assessment of a new silver sodium carboxymethylcellulose (AQUACEL® Ag BURN) glove in the management of partial thickness hand burns. Burns. 2012;38:1041–50.

85. Rahmanian-Schwarz A, Beiderwieden A, Willkomm LM, Amro A, Schaller H-E, Lotter O. A clinical evaluation of Biobrane and Suprathel in acute burns and reconstructive surgery. Burns. 2011;(37):1343–8.

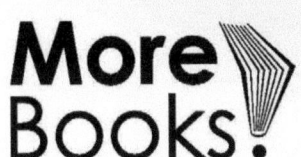
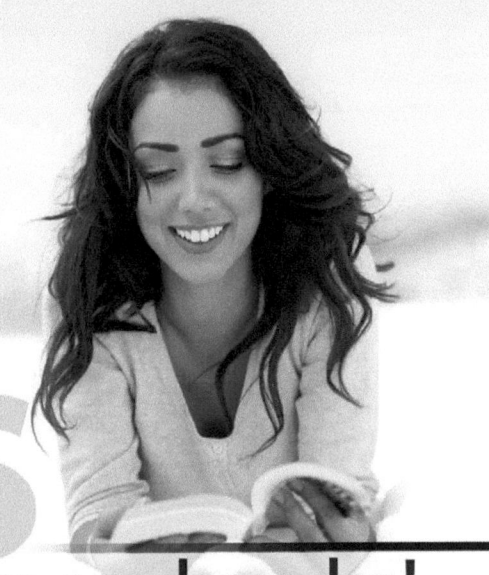
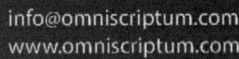
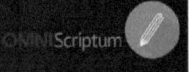

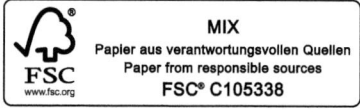

Printed by Books on Demand GmbH, Norderstedt / Germany